# OVERCOMING
# POOR
# POSTURE

## A SYSTEMATIC APPROACH TO REFINING
## YOUR POSTURE FOR HEALTH AND PERFORMANCE

**STEVEN LOW AND JARLO ILANO**

Published in Houston, Texas by Battle Ground Creative
First Edition

softcover ISBN: 978-1-947554-00-9
ebook ISBN: 978-1-947554-01-6

HEALTH & FITNESS / Exercise

Battle Ground Creative is a publishing company with an emphasis on helping first-time authors find their voice. Named after an obscure city in Washington State, we currently operate offices in Houston, Texas, and Princeton, New Jersey. For a complete title list and bulk order information, please visit www.battlegroundcreative.com.

The websites and references contained within this book are intended to serve as a resource with no guarantee expressed or implied as to the accuracy of their content.

Senior copyeditor: Jared Stump
Edited by: Jo Hsu
Proofreader: Andy Fossett
Cover design: Corinne Karl
Interior design and typeset: Katherine Lloyd
Models: Ryan Hurst and Alicia Nowak

Printed in the United States of America

# CONTENTS

## Chapter 1

# OVERVIEW AND PRACTICAL WAYS THIS BOOK CAN HELP YOU

Posture is one of the most misunderstood topics in both the fitness and medical worlds today. There are a lot of myths surrounding posture that are unhelpful and misleading, which results in a lot of wasted time and energy, as well as a lot of frustration. With all this misinformation, it is important to understand the mechanisms of posture within the body in order to look, feel, and perform better.

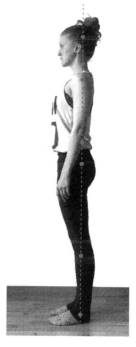

If there is one principle you must learn in fitness, it is that everything in the body reacts to the SAID principle—*specific adaptation to imposed demand*. The SAID principle shows us that when certain stimuli are applied to the body, it will adapt accordingly so that homeostasis is not disrupted. For example, if you perform resistance training with heavy weights, your body will react to this "imposed demand" with the "specific adaptation" of increasing bone density, increasing connective tissue integrity, increasing muscle mass, and gaining neurological adaptations to improve strength. Posture can be thought of as a similar process that responds to the imposed demands that you place on your body.

Traditionally, posture has been thought of as a static position. In fact, direct alignment of various bony landmarks on top of each other was considered to be "optimal" or "good" posture. These landmarks go from the ankles all the way up to the head. Linear positioning of these landmarks was often considered to be the best alignment. However, this has changed in recent years based on further research.

- Slightly anterior to the lateral malleolus.
- Slightly anterior to the axis of the knee.
- Slightly posterior to the axis of the hip (greater trochanter serves as a landmark).
- Bodies of the lumbar vertebrae.
- Bisecting the glenohumeral joint (head of the humerus, a.k.a. the shoulder).
- Bodies of most of the cervical vertebrae.
- Slightly posterior to the apex of the coronal suture (around the external occipital protuberance).

Posture is a very complex interplay between the neurological and musculoskeletal systems within the body, which all come together to make up a specific position. Some of the factors involved with modulating the interplay are habits, neurological reflexes, adaptations of the body, and time.[1] Let me give you some examples to help you understand these points better:

- Habits — *Habits* are easy to understand. We often sleep the same way, brush our teeth when we get up and when we sleep, and shower at particular times. There are many more examples throughout a typical day. In regard to posture and alignment, the habits of certain postures can also be ingrained in the body. Those who had parents who frequently told them to sit up straight or stand up straight will more likely default to that habit, which was ingrained in them from a young age. Those who had military training where they had to stand at attention will often default to those habits. Individuals who sit for very long periods of time or have desk jobs will tend to slump forward with a craned neck.

- **Neurological Reflexes** — Have you ever watched someone start to fall asleep in a car or on a plane? If they are sitting up in the chair and start to drift off to sleep, their body will naturally start to sway as their consciousness sinks deeper into sleep. Oftentimes you will see the body start to lean one way or the other and start to fall. Inexplicably, they may jerk upright without even waking up. This is a *neurological reflex* the body has within itself that does not require any conscious effort and that keeps the body upright.

- **Adaptations in the Body** — When maintaining physiological processes, the body tends to self-regulate to restore equilibrium. In particular, the body likes to be at the lowest possible state of energy, much like atoms or any other type of high(er) energy objects. Humans love to relax. The lowest possible energy state of the body is the parasympathetic nervous system state: eating, relaxing, lying down, and sleeping. Likewise, hunching over and sagging requires the least energy output from the body. When the muscles of the body are not active, we sag or round our backs while the bones and ligaments support our weight. This pursuit of "less effort" is one of the driving factors of slumping over when sitting.

- **Time** — *Time* is actually an interplay between habits and adaptations in the body. Specifically, in regards to posture, if you regularly sit at a computer desk or hunch over while studying, your body is going to try to minimize the work that it has to perform. Therefore, it will start tightening certain muscles and loosening other muscles to adapt to that specific posture. The time factor reminds you that it is not just specific exercises that affect your posture; everything else you do in the course of your day matters as well. Students and those with desk jobs often need to develop greater awareness than those with more activity in their lives.

As you can see, there is a lot of interplay between habits, neurological reflexes, and adaptations in the body that affects each individual's posture.

Since neurological reflexes are mostly out of our conscious control, we will focus on habit-building to correct any potential issues that require modification, and mindfulness to counter any potential issues with adaptations in the body. Habit-building and mindfulness will be critical for obtaining the benefits of posture and alignment.

If you have "poor" posture and you move your body into what is generally assumed to be "good" posture, you will find it uncomfortable. This is because your body has adapted to your poor posture, making it feel "normal" when it actually is not. Your default posture literally becomes a habit, just like smoking, binge eating, not flossing, or any other daily activity. It's very hard to break bad habits, especially if some time has passed and your body has adapted.

Subsequent chapters of this book will cover other discussions surrounding the history of postural correction, pain, the meaning of posture, and muscular tightness.

## CHAPTER SUMMARY

o   Your current posture is the result of your body's adaptations to the demands you place on it. Your body builds strength and flexibility where demand is placed on it, and loses strength and flexibility when no stressors are applied.

o   Posture is more than just a static position you hold throughout the day. It's the result of a variety of factors like habits (both good and bad), neurological reflexes, physical adaptations, and time.

## Chapter 2

# HOW POSTURAL TRAINING CAN IMPROVE YOUR LIFESTYLE

The benefits of good posture are tremendous. Evidence from various studies shows that improved posture can make you more powerful[2] and more confident.[3] This is common across the animal kingdom where different body postures play a role in social interaction and establishing hierarchy. While matters of social hierarchy are hotly debated amongst humans, the beneficial effects of good posture should not be ignored.

There are additional benefits to improved posture beyond just feeling more powerful and confident. The confidence gained from certain postures extends to self-perception in test-taking and interviewing.[4] Good posture can also boost testosterone,[5] decrease risk of developing illnesses,[6] and increase pain tolerance.[7] Neck angle can even affect cognitive processes in older adults.[8] All of these different benefits are related to what many would call good posture. However, that is not all that good posture can do.

A focus on posture puts the whole body into better alignment, which can help improve athletic performance and may decrease propensity for injuries. Also, it facilitates a more efficient breathing pattern. For example, just try taking nice, relaxed deep breaths while hunched over.

However, good posture or classifications of good posture are not rooted in reality. There is no such thing as a "proper" or "optimal" posture. Rather, it will be unique to each individual. This may seem counterintuitive, but it is not.

If poor posture were the cause of pain, would not those who had severe scoliosis be wracked with back pain? If posture were the cause of pain, wouldn't those confined to wheelchairs have more pain the longer they were in them? We know that those with severe scoliosis and those who are in wheelchairs are not always wracked with progressively-increasing lower back pain or any other type of pain. To the contrary, many of those with scoliosis or those in wheelchairs often have no back pain at all. This tells us that the body's posture cannot necessarily be classified as simply "good" or "bad."

Interestingly, studies have shown that the angle of pelvic tilt, lumbar lordosis, and thoracic kyphosis—the natural curve of the back—are not associated with increases in lower back pain.[9] Anterior pelvic tilt is commonly blamed for issues related to posture and lower back pain. This is false. It appears that posture itself is not involved in the development of back pain by itself. Rather, pain is caused by other factors. The conclusion of the Nourbakhsh study[10] gives us an indication of the factors involved in increased incidence of lower back pain:

> RESULTS: Among all the factors tested, endurance of the back extensor muscles had the highest association with LBP. Other factors such as the length of the back extensor muscles, and the strength of the hip flexor, hip adductor, and abdominal muscles also had a significant association with LBP.
>
> CONCLUSION: It appears that muscle endurance and weakness are associated with LBP and that structural factors such as the size of the lumbar lordosis, pelvic tilt, leg length discrepancy, and the length of abdominal, hamstring, and iliopsoas muscles are not associated with the occurrence of LBP.

The factors that lead to increased incidence of lower back pain are decreased muscle endurance and weakness rather than structural factors. This makes significantly more sense than posture or structural abnormalities such as the "angle of the back, pelvic tilt, leg length discrepancies, and length of certain muscles." Any posture that is difficult to sustain due to poor muscular endurance and/or weakness may end up causing discomfort and will likely result in pain.

This is not to say that bringing the body into a "better posture" is a bad thing or is not real. Bad posture is indeed rooted in reality—to an extent.

For instance, moving away from poor postures toward more powerful ones is "good" due to the psychological benefits mentioned in the previous section.

In similar scenarios, you can see that an extremely slumped posture or a posture that involves sitting for too long has detrimental effects on the body. In a study by Biswas entitled, "Sedentary Time and its Association with Risk for Disease Incidence, Mortality, and Hospitalization in Adults," researchers found that sitting increased the occurrence of mortality, cardiovascular disease, diabetes, and other maladies, regardless of whether a person exercised or not. Clearly, those who exercised more frequently decreased their risk, but sitting was still a factor in increased occurrences of the aforementioned conditions among those who spent extended periods of time sitting.

Paul Ingraham of *Pain Science* in his article "Does Posture Correction Matter?" ultimately uses the terminology *problem postures* instead of *bad posture*.[11] This is a more accurate indicator, because it shows that some postures may have more deleterious effects than others. Ingraham provides a separate but similar consideration to the issue of sitting postures, which may be hazardous to health by increasing the risk of all-cause mortality, disease, or arthritis. Some postures demand more endurance and strength from the various connective tissues, ligaments, and joints than others. This tends to be why we see a prevalence of neck pain among those who crane their neck and/or head forward and round their shoulders, as opposed to those who stand up straight. The cause is not necessarily those poor postures as much as it is the body's inability to effectively adapt to those positions.

In the majority of cases where "correcting posture" works—such as the traditional upper-crossed syndrome and the lower-crossed syndrome—the specific strength and endurance gains facilitate pain-reduction through increased load-tolerance, decreased instability, and decreased weakness. The pain from the "problematic posture" would disappear with increased strength and endurance regardless of whether or not the posture itself was changed.

It is important to realize that a key to resolving pain and discomfort is improving strength and endurance of the appropriate musculature. Changing a particular problematic posture is much more of a preventative measure that can fend off relapses.

Overall, postural alignment and the pursuit of its "ideal" engender a lot of arguments and controversy. From zealots who are adamant that there is only one perfect posture that will optimize everything in your life, to those who say that correcting specific postures means little to nothing in the grand scheme of things. Of course, like with other multifaceted and complex topics, the truth lies somewhere in between these two extremes.

As you will learn throughout this book, there is a chance that your quality of life will improve simply through the process of seeking to improve your posture. We have found that it is more about the process than the end goal. When you work through the strategies we present, you will learn your personal restrictions and weaknesses, thus allowing you to create a plan to compensate for them.

This will carry over into virtually every activity in your life, whether it is sitting and/or standing more comfortably at work, or achieving better form in your workouts and any sports you may play.

## CHAPTER SUMMARY

o   Improved alignment has positive effects on psychological well-being, breathing, energy conservation, and force production, which means that postural training can improve your physical performance as well.

o   Posture may not be the cause of pain, but changing your alignment can affect your pain through the strength, endurance, and mobility gained from postural training.

## FURTHER STUDY

- TED Talk from Amy Cuddy on how posture affects your confidence and self-perception: www.ted.com/talks/amy_cuddy_your _body_language_shapes_who_you_are

- Article from Todd Hargrove on the facets of good posture: www. bettermovement.org/blog/2010/three-essential-elements-of-good -posture

## Chapter 3

# THE CONNECTION BETWEEN POSTURE AND PAIN

P ain is a very complex topic. One of the first models of pain was the *gate control theory*. This theory quickly became outdated, and more models have begun to replace it. The two primary models are the *neuromatrix theory of pain*[12] and the *biopsychosocial model*[13], which attempt to accurately classify pain in the context of how it affects our daily lives.

The *biopsychosocial model of pain* asserts that there are biological, psychological, and social factors that influence pain within the body. These factors, along with other factors, may affect pain perception.

- Biological Factors — Pain from repetitive stress, injuries or trauma, nerve damage, illnesses, and similar phenomena that affect the body itself.
- Psychological Factors — The effect of emotions and thoughts, mood, attention, [lack of] sleep, [increased] anxiety, depression, fear, [lack of] trust, and other factors that may result in altered behaviors.
- Social Factors — Both biological and psychological inputs with pain can play a role in altering your social activities, relationships, work and occupation, and may lead to more isolation.
- Other Factors — These factors usually are external factors that alter any of the above three areas. Examples include medications, lack of available medical care, financial issues, and so on.

Similarly, the *neuromatrix theory of pain* looks specifically at the various biological and psychological factors in greater depth. The six general areas, verbatim, are:

- Cognitive Issues — Memories of past experiences, meaning (attributed to past experiences), and anxiety.
- Sensory Issues — The nociceptive (pain) inputs from cutaneous, visceral, and musculature senses.
- Emotional Issues — Limbic system and stress mechanisms. The limbic system regulates threat response in the brain.
- Pain Perception — Sensory, affective, and cognitive dimensions. How our brain interprets pain.
- Actions — Both voluntary and involuntary actions. Smash your knee and you may voluntarily or involuntarily rub it to alleviate some of the pain.
- Stress — The immune system, cortisol, and other stress hormones.

These two models represent factors that are known to contribute to pain. For example, stress, anxiety, and lack of sleep are known to effectively increase pain. Refraining from enjoyable activities also increases pain. Knowing these factors is important because you can take steps to avoid certain behaviors that may increase pain. You may also adopt certain behaviors—such as deep breathing, meditation, or other relaxation methods—that can help decrease pain.

One of the biggest areas in pain science that is now being explored is pain education. Among most patients and many health professionals, pain is one of the most misunderstood areas in rehabilitation. Likewise, it is easily misunderstood by the general public. Pain is very easily made into an object of fear, which leads to the catastrophizing of pain, framing it as something to avoid at all costs. This misconception negatively affects the rehabilitation process for patients and health professionals.

Reviews and studies have shown that pain education in regard to the above factors reduces pain directly (measured before and after pain education). Pain education has also been shown to reduce disability.[14] Dispelling what is called *fear* avoidance is critical in educating those with pain. Phrasing such as, "Pain is only in your brain," while somewhat true, do not actually help patients manage their pain. Conversely, this phrasing may lead to more detrimental behavior and increased pain over time. Instead, phrasing such as, "Hurt doesn't equal harm," "Stay active," and "Return to work as soon as possible" helps those with pain avoid developing behaviors that may have more detrimental psychological and social impact.[15]

Generally speaking, pain is a protective mechanism, not necessarily a symptom of damage.[16] The pathways of pain in the body can be over-sensitized to the point that normal positions or movements can sometimes elicit pain. This is one of the factors that can lead to the development of chronic pain. Thus, how one makes sense of their pain is an important factor for recovery.[17] Desensitizing the limbic and nervous systems with deep breathing, meditation techniques, and other relaxation techniques may also be useful, along with understanding the pain from a biological, psychological, and social perspective.[18]

For those who have "problematic postures with pain," it is important to be aware of the factors that influence pain and recovery. Not catastrophizing the pain, not avoiding various activities due to pain, and not changing your lifestyle around the pain are critical during a rehabilitation process.

The way we like to explain it to our patients/clients is by telling them to avoid aggravating exercises. Some exercises may cause pain, but they improve the performance and function of the injured area(s) after the exercise and/ or by the next session. Some exercises may not cause pain, but they definitely make the injury worse in terms of pain and function later on. Therefore, pain is not necessarily indicative of injury or harm. The key to rehabilitation progress is actively increasing strength, endurance, and stability in an area, with or without pain. As the process of rehabilitation continues, the pain will often go away.

Although painful exercises may not necessarily be detrimental, I like to avoid utilizing exercises that may cause pain during the rehabilitation process. The reason for this is that pain can negatively affect exercise technique due to compensations. It can also decrease the patients' motivation to get better, and it can negatively affect them psychologically and socially. Therefore, if there are solid rehabilitation exercises that can avoid pain, I will use those instead of the ones that elicit pain. Regardless of the route you take, pain education is necessary.

Because there are some instances when working through pain may be detrimental, I tend to recommend that painful exercises be used under the supervision of a rehabilitation professional. For instance, most patients or athletes do not have a good understanding of the types and volume of exercises required by the rehabilitation process. It is often the case that someone trying to utilize painful but beneficial exercises on their own may push too far and make an injury or dysfunction worse. Hence, it is important to get professional rehabilitation advice if you have an injury.

## PAIN AND MUSCULAR TIGHTNESS

Pain is often a prelude to muscular tightness. Another way of saying this is muscular tightness can lead to pain. They often tend to occur simultaneously, especially in the event of an acute injury. In terms of "problem postures," it is often the case that one will appear and then the other will follow. Whether pain precedes muscular tightness or vice versa does not matter in the grand scheme of things, as you still have to deal with both issues.

Generally, specific soft tissue work for the area in question should begin to help within two weeks or three to five sessions, if not resolve the pain completely. At the same time, this will give you enough time to remove the aggravating exercises from your routine and begin prehabilitation and isolation work to address the issue at hand. If the issue does not improve, there is likely something else going on that is interfering with improvements, or the fundamental issue itself is not being addressed. One example of an approach to pain and muscular tightness that is often misused is excessive foam rolling.

For instance, an athlete may experience pain and a tight back. Since the foam roller has been touted as a great way to loosen tight muscles, they may continuously use a foam roller or other massage-like implements to remove the knots and pain. Their back will improve for a period of time, but eventually stop improving. At this point, continuing to foam roll will not help; the tightness is actually being caused by something else.

The three most common causes of tightness in the back are pain, insta-bility, or weakness. You may have one of these things happening, two of them happening, or all of them happening at once. Take for example an ankle sprain: Pain and forceful movement to the end of your range of motion causes the muscles around the ankle to become tight as the body responds to the injury. A person who is double-jointed and hypermobile (such as con-tortionists or those with extreme flexibility) will have tight muscles because their body responds to the instability by tightening the muscles to prevent injury. If you have a weak or unstable back for whatever reason, your muscles may become tight to protect from injury.

In the case of foam rolling, you still have a tight back. This tightness could be caused by lingering pain from a previous injury. People with pain usually have significant tightness, which "magically" clears up as they heal from the injury. Instability could be another reason why your back is tight. Specific stability work for the spine may be the solution, rather than more foam rolling. Alternatively, your back could be weak and your muscles are tightening to protect it from injury. In that case, perform exercises to strengthen your back.

Exercises that are aimed at strengthening and stabilizing the back tend to clear up such instances of back pain and tightness. There are many dif-ferent types of physical therapy exercises that can be used to address these particular symptoms; these are classified as therapeutic exercise and neuro-muscular reeducation.

Additionally, more athletic-based exercises like low-weight, high-rep-etition kettlebell swings or reverse hyperextensions can be used in certain instances to alleviate back tightness and pain. This is helpful because ket-tlebell swings (with light weights) force your core muscles to stabilize your spine while simultaneously providing a stimulus for your back to become stronger under load. This corrects both instability and weakness simultane-ously. Over time, the pain will clear up and you will be left with a stronger, pain-free back. High-repetition reverse hyperextensions also provide the same benefits.

You should not attempt to resolve your back pain with kettlebell swings or reverse hyperextensions without consulting a medical professional. This information is intended to aid you in understanding these concepts, but should not serve as a substitute for medical advice. Generally speaking, if your injury gets worse or does not improve, stop exercising and consult a medical professional immediately.

This is also not to say that soft tissue work, massage, foam rolling, or myofascial work is useless. Far from it. What we are saying is you should wear your critical thinking hat in all circumstances. If an exercise is supposed to provide a certain result and it does not, you should ask yourself why this is the case. Understanding the underlying factors for each issue is important in order to produce effective bodily change.

To paraphrase the quote attributed to Albert Einstein, "The definition of insanity is doing the same thing repeatedly and expecting a different result."

Throwing your body at a foam roller in the hope that the tightness you are experiencing will dissipate when it repeatedly does not is insanity. While there is a time and a place for this, many athletes and trainers continue to utilize this type of work even when it does not produce results.

## THE BODY'S ADAPTIVE RESPONSES TO STRESS AND STRAIN OVER TIME

One excellent question that someone may ask when they experience pain is why "correcting their posture" is useful for rehabilitation. For example, many physical therapists often use postural correction as a useful part of a rehabilitation program for lower back and neck pain. Thus, the question, "If posture does not cause pain, why does correcting posture help solve pain?"

The answer is also counterintuitive. To understand this point, let's take a look at stretching as an example. Studies have shown us that stretching does not prevent injuries in athletic populations.[19] Although stretching prior to injury does not prevent injury, it is often used effectively in rehabilitation programs. Why is this?

Any nociceptive stimulus—pain—tends to lead to increased threat and therefore increased tension for many muscles in the body. For example, if you sprain your ankle, the muscles around your ankle will become much tighter. An increase in back pain will lead to tight muscles in the back. An increase in neck pain will lead to tight muscles in the neck. This is the body's adaptive response to a "threat." The response is aimed at reducing force output, movement, and range of motion in the injured area. The increased muscular tightness in a painful area will ensure that the injured person uses it less. Increased muscular tightness also diminishes the chances that a worse injury will occur. The body is all about self-preservation.

What is good for self-preservation is not necessarily good for health or athletic endeavors. Hence, stretching tight muscles can often be part of a program to help desensitize the threat response in the body, so that you can run again on that ankle or move your back and neck through the full range of motion.

At this point, you should see how postural correction can be used in response to an injury, though it is not part of the cause of the injury. In addition, I'd like to bring up a few things we discussed in chapter two: Strength and endurance are what resolve issues of pain, but moving away from the problematic posture will decrease stresses on various connective tissues, ligaments, and joints. These two factors are why "postural correction" exercises may be useful during a rehabilitation program. Increasing strength and endurance and decreasing stress while paying attention to how the body moves are all important.

One interesting observation I have made from reviewing various studies is that admonishing children and adolescents to straighten their backs does not work effectively.[20] This is true for children with hypermobility as well.[21] The reason that such commands are generally ineffective is because "straightening" one's back decreases the normal curvature of the spine (which is how it supports stress) and moves it toward end range, which may place excessive stress on the spine compared to normal ranges of motion.

## IMPLICATIONS FOR POSTURAL TRAINING

Throughout this book, we will present strategies for developing strength and mobility in order to improve your postural alignment. Rather than shooting for a perceived "ideal" posture, the exercises and recommendations will address your individual needs and concerns. The variety and efficiency of the various exercises, in addition to plans for implementation, will allow you to tailor the training for your unique goals.

We all know that decreasing pain and improving performance are very complicated issues; these topics literally fuel billions of dollars in products and services purporting to help. There are many factors that contribute to easing pain and bettering physical achievements. It's misleading for anyone to say they have the "one true way" of dealing with these concerns. Therefore, we are taking a pragmatic approach that is borne of our experiences with clients and patients, and informed by the latest evidence and research.

## CHAPTER SUMMARY

o   Pain is an incredibly complex topic that includes more than a direct cause and effect of bodily damage. Along with the biology of injury and trauma, other factors include the interplay of cognitive, sensory, and emotional issues, along with pain perception and stress. Variations occur both among individuals (when one person's reaction to an injurious event can be different from another) and also within ourselves (as when one incident can cause lasting pain, but a physically-equal experience elicits temporary pain).

o   Simply becoming better-educated about pain, and all of the factors that contribute to it, can diminish its effect on our daily lives and abilities. Understanding that pain is a protective mechanism and not a direct indicator of physical damage is a big factor in reducing suffering.

o   The development and sensation of muscular tightness often go hand in hand with pain, and improving tightness can decrease pain. However, there is more to addressing this tightness than just stretching and massage. It is important to assess and reassess your reactions to various methods.

o Postural work can assist in desensitizing our bodies' natural self-protective mechanisms.

## FURTHER STUDY

- Article from G. Lorimer Moseley on modern pain science: www.bodyinmind.org/resources/journal-articles/full-text-articles/reconceptualising-pain-according-to-modern-pain-science

- Article from Todd Hargrove on pain education's effects on lower back pain symptoms: www.bettermovement.org/2012/core-stabilization-versus-education-for-low-back-pain

## Chapter 4

# POSTURE IN REAL LIFE

Because studies have shown that certain postures do not necessarily correlate with pain, many health practitioners have shifted from using the term "posture" to using the term "alignment." These can be loaded words, but both essentially refer to having your joints aligned correctly.

To review, *posture* is defined as "a very complex interplay between the neurological and musculoskeletal systems within the body, which all come together to make up a specific position. Some of the factors involved with modulating the interplay are habits, neurological reflexes, adaptations of the body, and time."

> Posture is a very complex interplay between the neurological and musculoskeletal systems within the body, which all come together to make up a specific position. Some of the factors involved with modulating the interplay are habits, neurological reflexes, adaptations of the body, and time.

The *alignment* of the body is the relative positioning of the joints in relation to one another. In the context of everyday life and fitness, it is the positioning of limbs and joints such that the body is able to perform movements out of a certain posture. Obviously, this can be misconstrued into pseudoscientific nonsense very easily, so instead we should focus on the only part that makes sense. The part that makes sense is that different alignments facilitate movement. Hence, the title of this section.

For example, if you are an athlete who needs to lift something overhead such as in an overhead press or handstand pushup, there are definitely better "alignments" than others. Excessively rounded shoulders and head-forward alignment would put much unnecessary strain on the body and place the body in a suboptimal position for executing the movements. This would lead to poor performance. Likewise, what is traditionally assumed as "good posture," which is standing tall with shoulders back, is also not a good alignment for an overhead press or handstand pushup. These movements require a degree of protraction of the scapula—moving the shoulders forward into an optimal position.

Aligning the joints into a better position would allow more muscular force to be used, yielding both improved performance and less risk of injury. This is what is traditionally called technique. Therefore, both posture and alignment are best understood in terms of movement. Specifically, technique is the ability to move well from a certain posture (or alignment) that is good for the task at hand.

To expound on this: you are never really not moving at any point throughout the day. Even if you have a desk job, you constantly move into different positions. At times, you may slump over, crane your neck forward, round your shoulders, or turn to the side. It may seem like you are sitting still and straight. However, in reality, your body is in continual motion.

The key is not necessarily eliminating all of the different facets of sitting, although some may be worse than others. The key is finding and moving between positions that do not place excessive strain on the body, which may lead to detrimental effects down the road. Being rigid and sticking in a position that is assumed to be "good posture" or "good alignment" is also not good. We may shift into "poor posture" at times because we want to be able to move and stretch out. Our bodies are meant to move.

Sitting up in your chair will often bring you into better alignment than slumping forward with rounded shoulders and a craned neck. It will also put less (potentially problematic) strain on your back, neck, and shoulders. But, is sitting up in the nice, straight, and rigid position going to be good long term? No! You want to be able to move effectively and efficiently from that position. Can you move well out of it? Can you rotate to grab things to your side without bending over and twisting (which is a risk factor for back injuries)? Can you reach for something without craning your neck and shoulders for it?

Think about posture and alignment in the context of moving well and the ability to adapt effectively to your environment while avoiding injury-prone positioning. That should give you a better idea of where we are coming from and where we are trying to go.

## CHAPTER SUMMARY

o  What one may refer to as "good posture" is better thought of as "proper alignment" for a task or technique. There is no alignment that fits all situations. Reframing it in this manner shifts your thinking from one ideal posture to something that is more personalized to you. Being able to effectively move into and out of various improved alignments will help your body function better on a daily basis.

## FURTHER STUDY

- Article from Anthony Mychal on postural alignment's role in athleticism: www.anthonymychal.com/muscle-imbalances -generators-connectedness-and-3-tips-to-clean-up-athleticism

- Article from Monika Schloder on the role of posture in sports performance: www.coachingbest.com/the-importance-of-posture -in-sports-performance

- Article from Andrew Hamilton on the importance of posture for athletes: www.peakendurancesport.com/endurance-injuries-and -health/endurance-health-and-lifestyle/components-posture- importance-athletes

## Chapter 5

# PRACTICAL STEPS TO IMPROVING POSTURE

We will now dive into the practical side of this book; namely, outlining strategies for corrective exercise, habit formation, and mindset reframing. These will assist you in finding and improving your body's optimal posture.

The term *corrective exercise* generally refers to specific movements for those with specific restrictions. It shouldn't imply that these exercises are the only way to deal with impediments and limitations. The exercises we've chosen to share here have proven to be efficient and useful for our patients and clients over the years. Most of these exercises require no equipment and can be performed anywhere.

Habits and the processes of personal change are incredibly important topics in any discussion of self-transformation. Without an understanding of the fundamentals of how habits are developed and maintained, any program can be derailed by a lack of interest or burnout. Consistent effort, over time, is one of the cornerstones of physical change, and everything you can do to encourage this is beneficial.

In addition to physical training and changes in habits, mental work is necessary to align your goals with your actions and expectations. Your mindsets can either be positive or negative. More specifically, your mindset can foster growth and advancement, or it can be fixed and rigid. It is absolutely necessary to believe that you can get better, given consistent effort and time. If you don't believe this, you can inadvertently end up sabotaging your efforts to change.

Let's begin by discussing the foundations of the corrective exercises we've chosen for this book, and then move to the habits and mental framework needed to utilize them consistently for the long haul.

## FUNDAMENTALS OF THE PHYSICAL RESTRICTIONS OF POSTURE

The terms *Upper crossed syndrome* (UCS) and *lower crossed syndrome* (LCS) come from the work of Vladimir Janda, circa 1987-1988.[22] Janda's work describes a pattern of weakness and tightness in the upper and lower body that is common within desk job culture.

For example, UCS and LCS would typically exhibit these common features:

- Upper Crossed Syndrome – Head-forward Posture: weak neck flexors, weak scapular retractors, tight upper cervical muscles/suboccipitals, tight chest pec/pec minor/rounded shoulders.
- Lower Crossed Syndrome – Anterior Pelvic Tilt: weak glutes, weak abs, tight hip flexors, tight back.

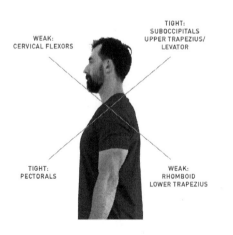
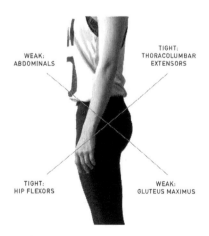

Upper Crossed Syndrome          Lower Crossed Syndrome

In light of new research, we now know that tight muscles are not necessarily strong, and we know that loose or lengthened muscles are not necessarily weak. Tight muscles can be weak, and lengthened muscles can be strong. This throws a wrench into UCS and LCS in terms of using them to correct posture to improve pain and/or performance.

Instead, UCS and LCS postures need to be thought of as symptoms of the actual, underlying cause. They arise from a large number of habits, neurological reflexes, adaptations, and time accumulated in those positions. Desk jobs and studying have effectively become a "culture." It is this culture that shapes the postural appearance of what is traditionally termed UCS and LCS, which are simply symptoms of the cultural stresses accumulated by the body over time.

The body likes to be as energy-efficient as possible for the task at hand. Sitting with your neck craned forward and shoulders rounded is actually the most efficient posture for that position. This is why the body always tends toward that particular state when you remain in this position for an extended period of time. Unfortunately, this posture tends to have negative long-term effects on the body.

While such a posture may not be the particular cause of pain, the state of having your neck craned forward and your shoulders rounded has shown some evidence of decreased function on outcome measures such as the Neck Disability Index (NDI), though the NDI does not measure psychological or social factors.[23] The NDI not only looks at pain, but also functional movement throughout daily life; for example, the ability to do personal care like washing, lifting, reading, evaluating your headaches, concentrating, working, driving, sleeping, and enjoying recreation. Therefore, even though something like UCS does not exist as purported, there is evidence to suggest that the head-forward/rounded shoulders posture may cause some issues.

Indeed, because this posture is efficient, it may lead to particular weaknesses and lack of endurance in specific muscles without exercise. This is why this posture sometimes causes pain or discomfort. Thus, the benefits from any corrective exercises stem from the exercises and movements themselves. It is not that there are necessarily any imbalances with tight/loose muscles or strong/weak muscles, but overall disuse that contributes to extensive weakness, instability, or loss of endurance.

While UCS and LCS do not exist as purported, the descriptions of the postures can still be useful heuristics for examining some of the common issues among students and desk job culture. Strengthening and stabilizing these areas can help reduce these effects in particular. However, most of the actual correction is going to come from mindfulness and sustained habits.

To give you an accurate analogy, any stretching and exercise is like a bandage. It will help cover a wound and protect it, but the real healing comes from your body engaging in the healing process. Mindfulness and sustained habits that aid this process are key. This knowledge will guide us in the next few chapters, as we look at various range-of-motion, strengthening, and stability exercises.

## CHAPTER SUMMARY

o *Corrective exercise* refers to the specific strengthening, flexibility, and body-awareness work that is best for you. There are common patterns like those identified in the UCS and LCS models, as well as individual issues that you will discover for yourself when you begin using the exercises we share in this book.

o Certain exercises are only a portion of the changes you must make in how you hold yourself as you move throughout your day. Mindfulness and sustained habits are additional key components of overcoming poor posture and will require just as much work.

## FURTHER STUDY

- *Neanderthal No More*, five-part series from Eric Cressey and Mike Robertson that is billed "the complete guide to fixing your caveman posture":

- o www.t-nation.com/training/neanderthal-no-more-1
- o www.t-nation.com/training/neanderthal-no-more-2
- o www.t-nation.com/training/neanderthal-no-more-3
- o www.t-nation.com/workouts/neanderthal-no-more-4
- o www.t-nation.com/workouts/neanderthal-no-more-5

- Article from Bret Contreras on fixing anterior pelvic tilt: www.t-nation.com/training/dont-be-like-donald-duck

- Three-part series from Dean Somerset on the thoracic spine:
  - o www.deansomerset.com/all-things-thoracic-spine-part-1-functional-anatomy
  - o www.deansomerset.com/all-things-thoracic-spine-part-two-assessments-and-figuring-it-all-out
  - o www.deansomerset.com/all-things-thoracic-spine-part-3-corrective-strategies

- Four articles from Anthony Mychal on strength imbalances:
  - o www.anthonymychal.com/can-correcting-strength-imbalances-cause-injury-part-i
  - o www.anthonymychal.com/can-correcting-strength-imbalances-cause-injury-part-ii
  - o www.anthonymychal.com/can-correcting-strength-imbalances-cause-injury-part-iii
  - o www.anthonymychal.com/strength-imbalances-put-to-rest-why-great-athletes-are-imbalanced

- *Shoes, Sitting, and Lower Body Dysfunctions*, article from Steven Low: www.stevenlow.org/shoes-sitting-and-lower-body-dysfunctions

## Chapter 6

# CORRECTIVE EXERCISES FOR YOUR POSTURE

We have categorized these exercises into different groups to assist you in choosing what is best for you based on your individual needs and goals. In the appendix of this book, you will find sample plans that you can choose from as well.

Mobility and stability exercises improve your range of motion through either dynamic movement or static holds. These two types of exercises are paired together because your goal should be to maintain control through your entire range of motion and these exercises emphasize that.

The strength and endurance exercises include movements you are likely familiar with and focus on the musculature that contributes most to your ability to maintain good postural positioning in your daily and recreational activities.

Resets are movements/postures that are exaggerations of the postural positions with which most people have difficulty. Some positions can be difficult to attain due to restrictions in strength and/or flexibility, and also due to limitations in body awareness. Simply put, your body does not "know" that it can obtain and hold the position. Thus, practicing these movements will aid you in developing improved proprioceptive senses.

**DISCLAIMER:** *Do not attempt any type of exercise or program until you are first cleared by the appropriate medical professional. Some exercises listed may be contraindicated for specific conditions. Hence,* *performing any of these exercises may lead to more serious injuries. Any information contained herein is for informational purposes only. All exercises are performed at your own risk. The authors, publisher, and any agents of this book will not be responsible for any injuries.*

## EXERCISES FOR MOBILITY/STABILITY

### *Full Range of Motion in Flexion and Extension*

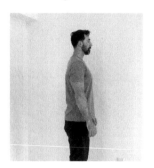 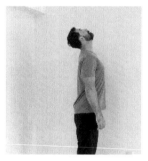 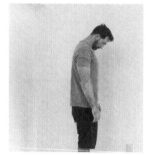

Slowly move your head and contract the back of your neck muscles. Continue until your neck is fully extended. Slowly bend your neck from this position and come down until your chin touches your chest.

You may experience stretching of the front of the neck while extending the neck back and looking up, and you may experience some stretching in the back of the neck while moving the head forward and looking down. This is normal.

Those who have had head-forward posture for a while may experience discomfort moving into ranges of motion they have not used in a while. Take it slow and be patient. If a particular range feels too uncomfortable, back off and move within a comfortable range of motion for a few repetitions before attempting it again.

#### *Chin Tucks*

This exercise slightly strengthens and increases endurance in the deep flexors of the neck while simultaneously lengthening the muscles on the back of the neck. In head-forward posture, the muscles of the deep flexors and the back of the head can often become weak. Thus, this exercise is one of the first steps to begin activating and moving the neck well once again.

First, place your fingers on the back of your neck and slowly move them up your neck until you feel a bump that is a few inches above your hair line. This bump is called the *external occipital protuberance*. This bony landmark can be used to assess correct positioning while performing these exercises.

If you are a beginner, you should know that there are multiple variations of chin tucks. The first variation is performed in the supine position, which is lying down on your back.

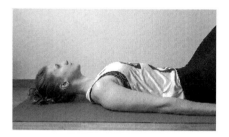 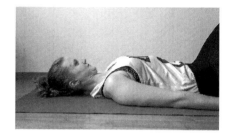

To perform this variation of chin tucks, lie on your back on a flat, firm surface (a floor or firm mattress works fine). Slowly retract your chin so that your head moves backward. If you have significant "head-forward" posture your chin should begin to tuck in, hence the name of the exercise. It may feel like the skin on your neck is bunching up and forming a double chin, which means you are in the correct position. Hold for five to ten seconds.

During this exercise, your external occipital protuberance should come back and press down into the into the floor (or a pillow if the surface is too hard). You should also feel the muscles on the front of your neck begin to contract, and the muscles on the back of your neck begin to lengthen and potentially stretch. This is normal.

If you have had head-forward posture for many months or years, this movement may feel stiff and difficult. This is because you have likely not moved into this range of motion for some time, and is therefore normal. Take it slow and allow your neck to acclimate to the movement over time.

The second variation of chin tucks is performed while standing, often with the assistance of a wall.

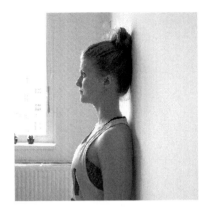 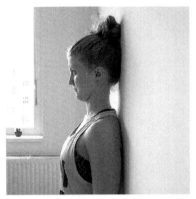

First, place your back flat against a wall (or the corner of a wall). Position your feet so that your heels are approximately an inch or two away from the wall. There should be a natural curve in your spine so that your butt and the area between your shoulder blades is against the wall, but your lower back is not against the wall. If you have head-forward posture, there is a good chance your head will pull forward away from the wall in this position.

From this standing position with your back against the wall, slowly perform the chin tuck motion. Your chin will come back toward your body, thus resulting in contraction of your front neck flexor muscles and lengthening of the back of your neck muscles. Continue to slowly bring the chin tuck back until the back of your head touches the wall. At this point, it should be your external occipital protuberance that touches the back of the wall. If you have normal neck lordotic curve, the rest of your neck and head should not be touching the wall. Hold this position for five to ten seconds.

After you repeat this exercise for five to ten repetitions, you can progress to standing away from the wall. However, you should only do this when you come to an understanding of how this movement feels at end range. Your goal should be getting accustomed to moving your neck through the full range of motion and acquire body awareness through said range of motion. You may feel a stretching sensation on the back and side of your neck as you do this.

If you have had head-forward posture for many months or years, this movement may feel stiff and difficult. This is probably normal if you have not moved into this range of motion for some time. Take it slow and allow your neck to acclimate to the movement over time. You may not be able to bring your head back against the wall for the first session or even the first few sessions. Generally speaking, the range of motion will come slowly over time. Avoid pushing through any pain. There will be some slight discomfort or stretching feeling, but there should not be any type of pain.

### Chin Tuck with Side Bending Movement

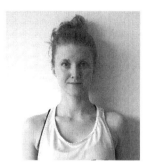 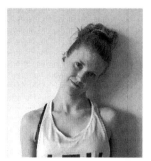 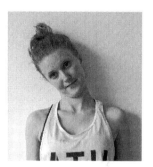

*Chin tucks with side bending movement* are performed from the initial chin tuck position. Here are the basic instructions: Stand with your back against the wall, bring your chin back so that your external occipital protuberance comes back to the wall.

From this position with the back of your head against wall, slowly bend your head from side to side while keeping your head facing straight forward. You may feel a stretching feeling in the back of your neck, but once you get used to the chin tuck movement this will go away. When you begin side bending with the chin tuck you will often feel an increased stretching feeling opposite from the direction in which you are bending your neck. These are your scalene muscles stretching throughout the movement.

Over time, you will want to slowly work toward tilting your head 30 to 45 degrees in either direction. This may take multiple sessions or weeks depending on how long you have had head-forward posture.

The goal is to become comfortable with multiple planes of motion. Our necks have the ability to move well, but we often do not take full advantage of this due to our "desk job" culture. This leads to stiffness, lack of range of motion, lack of endurance, and weakness. These exercises are progressed with different movements to help you acclimate to moving well once again.

In most cases, you will find that your chin tucks become significantly easier as you move back and forth within this movement. The reason for this is because the chin tuck pattern is best performed in a variety of ways. It is very difficult to become comfortable with only a single plane of motion. Once you begin adding another plane of motion to chin tucks, you'll notice that your restrictions will decrease. This will make chin tucks much easier and more comfortable to perform.

One of the major issues with many "posture" programs is that they only focus on getting your body into a specific postural position. Many programs only use chin tucks to get your body into this position. As you now know, this is an inefficient and non-productive way to approach moving your body away from problematic postures. It is more effective to move away from particular postures with movements like chin tucks and to then progress into a wider variety of movements. This will make it much easier and more comfortable to maintain non-problematic postures, which your body will begin to naturally default to over its former postures.

You can progress to performing this exercise without wall assistance as soon as you are comfortable with the positioning.

### Chin Tuck with Rotation Movement

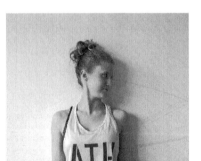 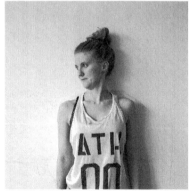

*Chin tucks with rotation movement* are performed from the initial chin tuck position. To reiterate the basic instructions: Stand with your back against the wall, bring your chin back so that your external occipital protuberance comes back to the wall.

From this position, with the back of your head against wall, begin to slowly look to your left and to your right. Keep your head and eyes level when looking back and forth. You will likely begin to feel a stretching sensation on portions of your neck, and activation of the muscles on the other side of the neck. This will happen with both the muscles in the front, side, and back of your neck. As you become more comfortable with the movement, continue to increase your range of motion.

Over time, you will want to slowly work toward being able to look fully to the right and fully to the left. This may take multiple sessions or weeks depending on how long you have had head-forward posture.

As with the side bending movement, your goal is to become more comfortable with multiple planes of motion. You should find that simple movements like chin tucks become much easier. Adding this movement to your chin tucks will make all your other movements more comfortable, and you'll revert to problematic postures less often. See the previous section for more details on the reasoning behind this.

You can progress to performing this exercise without wall assistance as soon as you are comfortable with the positioning.

### *45-degree Chin Tucks*

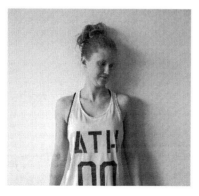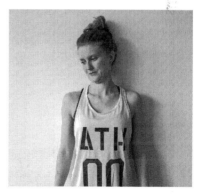

*45-degree chin tucks* are performed from the initial chin tuck position. To reiterate the basic instructions: Stand with your back against the wall, bring your chin back so that your external occipital protuberance comes back to the wall.

This movement is different from traditional chin tucks, in that you will add some rotation so that you are looking 45 degrees to your left or to your right. From there, you are going to bring your chin forward, in a similar manner to head-forward posture. Next, slowly bring your neck back.

This movement is a "test piece" type of movement because it shows that you are now able to move well in multi-plane movements. As you get more comfortable with movements like these, you can start bending, rotating, and moving your head in different planes of movement at the same time. Go slowly and be aware of tightness and restrictions as you move. Play a bit with the range in order to loosen up those restrictions.

*Supine Hooklying Anterior and Posterior Pelvic Tilt*

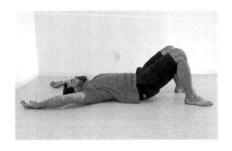

Posterior Pelvic Tilt

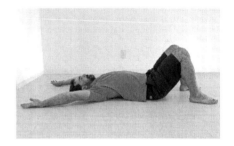

Anterior Pelvic Tilt

This exercise is mainly here to cultivate awareness of pelvis orientation in space. Those with lower back pain or discomfort often have very poor proprioceptive and kinesthetic awareness of the back and pelvis in relation to one another. These individuals' movements become much more gross motor and "blocky" because the body does not want to do anything that can cause pain. With back pain in particular, there can be delayed activation of some of the core musculature such as the transverse abdominals.

Begin by lying on your back on the floor or a bed with your knees bent and your feet flat on the ground. There are a couple cues for understanding posterior pelvic tilt in this position. Some cues may not work for you, so find one that does work. The first cue is to flatten your back flat against the floor. The second is to squeeze your glutes and bring your belly button to the floor. The third is to simply round your back.

To perform the anterior pelvic tilt, you want to move the opposite way and create space between your lower back and the ground. The first cue is to arch your back away from the floor. This will make your back extend and your pelvis tilt away from you. The second cue is to use your hip flexors to pull your pelvis toward your legs and tilt your belly button away from you. The third cue is to simply arch your back upward.

Generally speaking, one position is usually more difficult for people to learn than the other. Prolonged sitting in our culture causes our bodies to be more accustomed to anterior pelvic tilt over posterior pelvic tilt. Some individuals, especially those with previous back injuries or lower back pain, may struggle with both of these movements.

Two bonus movements you can perform are side bends in this position. First, tilt your right hip up toward the right side of the rib cage. Then, straighten your torso before tilting your left hip up toward your left rib cage.

Learning how to move your pelvis comfortably in all of these positions, including the bonus movements, is the key to dissociating your pelvis from your core. This is integral to learning how to move well again. Studies tell us that the static positions of anterior or posterior pelvic tilt are not associated with lower back pain. However, learning how to move your body more effectively will pay dividends in the long run.

### Quadruped Cat Camel

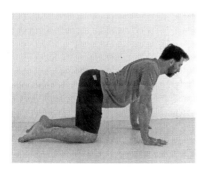 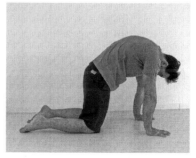

For *quadruped cat camel,* begin on your hands and knees. Your shoulder and hip angles should be 90 degrees. To move into the "cat" position from a straight back, anteriorly tilt your pelvis slowly, bringing your belly button closer to the floor. This will cause your back to arch. One cue that can help you achieve this position is to look up slowly while you arch your back. Pause at the end of the movement before slowly beginning to move into the "camel" position. You will move through the neutral position. Aim to move your back as high as possible, posteriorly tilting your pelvis and drawing your belly button up toward the ceiling. The head movement that may accompany this is bringing your chin to your chest. Pause at the end of the movement and repeat as needed.

This exercise progresses the supine hooklying anterior and posterior pelvic tilt into another position.

### Quadruped Spinal Circles

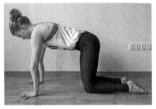 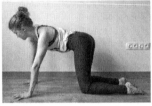 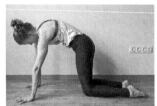

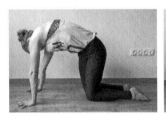 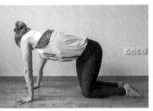 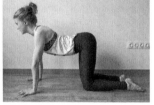

Just as for cat/camel, begin on your hands and knees with your shoulders, elbows and hands lined up at a 90-degree angle. Your hips and knees should be aligned at this angle as well. Begin by going into the "camel" position and then move your spine to one side and work down to the "cat" position on that side. You will have made a half circle. Continue on making a full circle back to the "camel" position. Think of moving your chest in as big of a circle as possible as you complete this movement.

This is consistently difficult for many people when they first attempt it. Many people experience a lot of difficulty moving their spine independently of their shoulders and hips, which makes this an especially important movement.

### Quadruped Spinal Side Bending (Wag Tail)

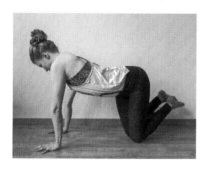 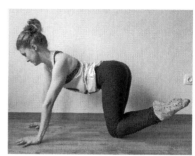

This exercise, which emphasizes spinal side bending, is also performed on your hands and knees. Begin in a "neutral" position, with your back flat (like a table top). Next, bring your knees together to touch and lift your feet up. Keep your back flat and rotate around your knees by bending your spine to one side and then the other.

Once you are comfortable with this, it is very useful to do this movement with a rounded back (camel position) and an arched back (cat position) for different effects.

### Elbows-on-Wall Thoracic Extension

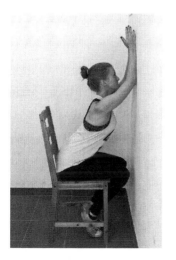 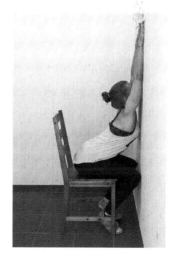

Good extension (or backward bending) in the thoracic spine is essential for changing posture. It is the opposite of the hunched-over position that most people picture when they think of "poor posture."

Begin by sitting down, facing a wall, with a chair far enough away so you can lean with your forearms flat against the wall while keeping your back flat. Now, use the positioning of your elbows as leverage to scoop your chest forward and up (toward the wall). It is helpful to inhale as you do this. Hold for a few seconds and then relax back to the starting position.

### Prone Extension Press

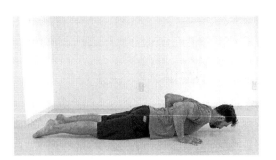 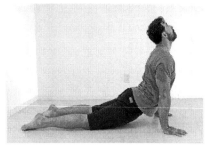

Note: Do not perform this exercise if you have a lower back injury. Prone extension may help some lower back injuries, but it is contra-indicated for other back injuries and may make them significantly worse.

*Prone extension* is very similar to the elbow prone neck extension exercise, except there is movement involved. For prone extension, begin with your elbows resting on a soft, flat surface. Your back should naturally be arched with your stomach and legs on the floor, mattress, or other surface. Slowly push through your hands to raise your chest up. If you are able, push through your hands until your elbows are fully straight. Then, slowly lower back down to your elbows. For a bonus movement, attempt to bend your legs (so that your heels touch your butt) while keeping your elbows straight. This will help stretch out your hip flexors and quads.

Most people who work at a desk or spend extended periods of time studying, driving, or performing sitting-related tasks are in a position where their heads are forward and their shoulders/back are rounded for the majority of the day. This can cause the muscles in the front of your body (quads, hip flexors, and abdominals) to grow tight. To counteract this, move your spine into extension.

You may find that you are too weak to push your elbows to the top of the prone position. If this is the case, one substitution involves beginning with your hands on the floor in the bottom of the pushup position. Next, push through your hands so that your arms straighten. Instead of keeping your body straight (like a pushup), allow your back to arch and your hip flexors and abdominals to stretch until your arms are straight. If you have access to an incline table, you may want to utilize it to make the movement easier. Alternatively, you can ask someone to assist you if necessary.

The downward dog to upward dog position (commonly used in yoga) is also a good alternative if you prefer.

This book will not cover gymnastics bridges, but they can also be an effective tool for stretching your back into extension as a higher-level progression.

## Segmental Rolling

*Segmental rolling* is one of my favorite exercises to promote stability, decrease tightness, and increase overall comfort and well-being in patients and athletes alike. Infants naturally learn this movement at about six months of age as they learn to roll over, and the pattern is associated with various proprioceptive neuromuscular facilitation patterns. Basically, rolling is one of the most important patterns to learn. It coordinates trunk and limb movement and effectively activates the small stabilizing muscles in your spine. If I could only recommend a single exercise for those with tight backs and back pain, this would be my exercise of choice.

There are eight different rolls that you can perform with segmental rolling. Four are supine on your back with your body facing up, and four are prone on your front with your body facing the floor. Each movement begins with a different limb. I am going to teach them to you as "limb rolls" to make it easier to understand, rather than facing up or facing down. It is easier to go limb by limb rather than continually switching back and forth between each of them.

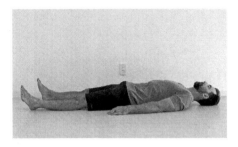 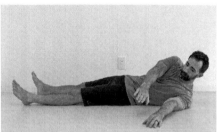

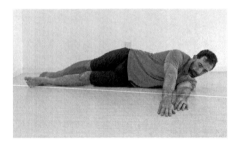 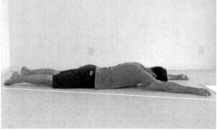

**Facing Up, Right Arm Roll** — Begin with your body facing up and your arms and legs in a slight X shape. Bring your right arm across your body, lifting your right shoulder off the ground. Your abdominal muscles should begin firing as you bring your arm across your body. Continue to bring your arm all the way across your body, and allow your torso to roll with you. As you begin to turn over onto your stomach, do not bring your right leg with you. Instead, allow the rolling movement to bring it along. You should now find yourself on your stomach in a prone position. Adjust your limb positioning back into the slight X shape while remaining on your stomach.

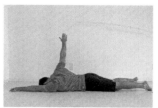 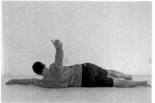 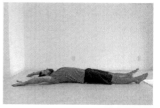

**Facing Down, Right Arm Roll** — Begin with your body facing down and your arms and legs in a slight X shape. Bring your right arm backward across your body, lifting your right shoulder off the ground. Your right shoulder blade should pull back as you do this, and your back muscles will activate as your arm moves backward over your body. Continue to bring your arm toward the ground and allow your torso to roll with you. As you begin to turn over onto your back, do not bring your right leg with you. Instead, allow the rolling movement to bring it along. You should now find yourself on your back in a supine position. Adjust your limb positioning back into the slight X shape while remaining on your back.

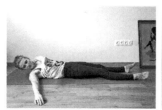 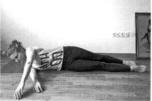 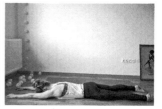

**Facing Up, Left Arm Roll** — Begin with your body facing up and your arms and legs in a slight X shape. Bring your left arm across your body, lifting your left shoulder off the ground. Your abdominal muscles should begin firing as you bring your arm across your body. Continue to bring your arm all the way across your body and allow your torso to roll with you. As you begin to turn over onto your stomach, do not bring your left leg with you. Instead, allow the rolling movement to bring it along. You should now find yourself on your stomach in a prone position. Adjust your limb positioning back into the slight X shape while remaining on your stomach.

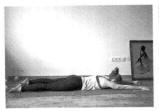 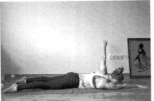 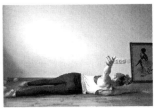

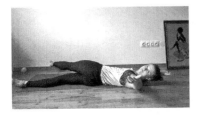 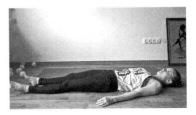

**Facing Down, Left Arm Roll** — Begin with your body facing down and your arms and legs in a slight X shape. Bring your left arm backward across your body, lifting your left shoulder off the ground. Your left shoulder blade should pull back as you do this, and your back muscles will activate as your arm moves backward over your body. Continue to bring your arm all the way across your body and allow your torso to roll with you. As you begin to turn over onto your back, do not bring your left leg with you. Instead, allow the rolling movement to bring it along. You should now find yourself on your back in a supine position. Adjust your limb positioning back into the slight X shape while remaining on your back.

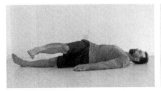 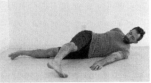 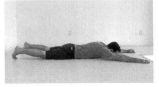

**Facing Up, Right Leg Roll** — Begin with your body facing up and your arms and legs in a slight X shape. Bring your right leg across your body, lifting your right hip off the ground. Your abdominal muscles should begin firing as you bring your leg across your body. Continue to bring your leg all the way across your body and allow your torso to roll with you. As you begin to turn over onto your stomach, do not bring your right arm with you. Instead, allow the rolling movement to bring it along. You should now find yourself on your stomach in a prone position. Adjust your limb positioning back into the slight X shape while remaining on your stomach.

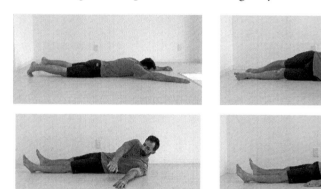

**Facing Down, Right Leg Roll** — Begin with your body facing down and your arms and legs in a slight X shape. Bring your right leg backward across your body, lifting your right hip off the ground. Your back muscles will activate as your leg moves backward over your body. Continue to bring your leg all the way across your body and allow your torso to roll with you. As you begin to turn over onto your back, do not bring your right arm with you. Instead, allow the rolling movement to bring it along. You should now find yourself on your back in a supine position. Adjust your limb positioning back into the slight X shape while remaining on your back.

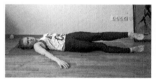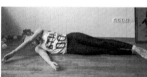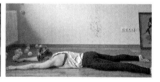

**Facing Up, Left Leg Roll** — Begin with your body facing up and your arms and legs in a slight X shape. Bring your left leg across your body, lifting your left hip off the ground. Your abdominal muscles should begin firing as you bring the leg across your body. Continue to bring your leg all the way across your body and allow your torso to roll with you. As you begin to turn over onto your stomach, do not bring your left arm with you. Instead, allow the rolling movement to bring it along. You should now find yourself on your stomach in a prone position. Adjust your limb positioning back into the slight X shape while remaining on your stomach.

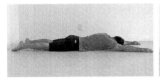 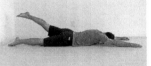 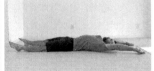

**Facing Down, Left Leg Roll** — Begin with your body facing down with your arms and legs in a slight X shape. Bring your left leg backward across your body, lifting your left hip off the ground. Your back muscles will activate as your leg moves backward over your body. Continue to bring your leg all the way across your body and allow your torso to roll with you. As you begin to turn over onto your back, do not bring your left arm with you. Instead, allow the rolling movement to bring it along. You should now find yourself on your back in a supine position. Adjust your limb positioning back into the slight X shape while remaining on your back.

It may take a significant amount of time to perform a few sets of all of the different segmental rolling variations with multiple repetitions in each set. However, after you begin to do them you will not want to stop. They will make the muscles in your shoulders, hips, back, and torso feel much more comfortable and stable. This is one exercise you can perform through-out the day for lasting benefits with little fatigue.

### *Hip Flexor Stretch (Couch or Wall)*

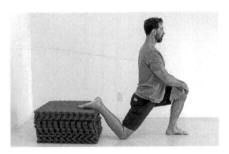

Set yourself up for this exercise by beginning in a lunge position, with your back to the wall or a couch. Next, bend your back leg so that your toes or the top of your foot is up against the wall. Scoot back so that your heel is as close to your butt as possible. You can now set up for the lunge position. Bring your upper body into an upright position and begin to lunge forward as you squeeze your glute muscles (found in the back of your leg). You should feel a stretch in your hip flexors and quadriceps during this movement. Hold for ten to thirty seconds. Slowly back out of the lunge and repeat with the opposite side of your body.

If you are new to this exercise, it can be difficult to maintain your balance. Therefore, you may desire to use chairs or other stable objects for assistance. This is fine for beginners, but you will ultimately want to work toward eliminating any form of assistance as you progress.

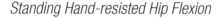

### Standing Hand-resisted Hip Flexion

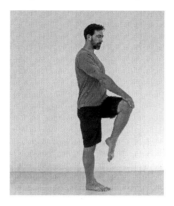

For this exercise, start by standing near a wall or other stable object. Pick one leg to raise and one leg to stand on (for the sake of this example, I am utilizing the left leg to raise and the right leg to stand on). Place your left hand on the wall or stable object for balance. Next, slowly lift your left leg and bend your knee up while standing on your right leg. As your knee approaches the height of your hips, place your right hand across your body and push down on your left knee. As you push down with your right hand, your left knee should push up into your right hand. Hold this position for five to ten seconds. Slowly take your right hand off of your left knee and lower your left leg to the ground. Repeat on the opposite side.

*Standing hand-resisted hip flexion* is one of the best exercises to get a handle on pelvis positioning while standing. During the exercise, your standing leg glute will contract, your pelvis will rotate to a neutral position, your hip flexors and abdominals will contract on the leg that is being lifted, and your core will stabilize the axial rotation due to the pressure from your leg.

Once you bring your leg down and repeat this exercise a few times on each side, you should have a better sense of your pelvis position. This exercise will also give you a feel for contracting various muscles around your pelvis, which include your glutes, hip flexors, and abdominals.

As you progress with this exercise, your first step should be moving away from the wall so your body learns to balance without assistance.

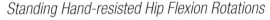

*Standing Hand-resisted Hip Flexion Rotations*

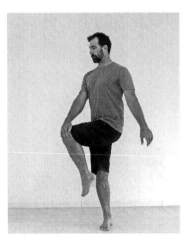

*Standing hand-resisted hip flexion rotations* are a more difficult progression of the previous exercise.

For this exercise, first stand by a wall or other stable object. Pick one leg to raise and one leg to stand on (for the sake of this example, I am utilizing the left leg to raise and the right leg to stand on). Place your left hand on the wall or stable object for balance. Next, slowly lift your left leg and bend your knee up while standing on your right leg. As your knee approaches the height of your hips, place your right hand across your body and push down on your left knee. As you push down with your right hand, your left knee should push up into your right hand.

Once you perform this, keep your left leg knee-level and slowly rotate your body to the left. Keep your hand on the wall if needed for balance, but do not use it to pull or turn your body. Your right hip muscles should be performing the work. Continue to slowly rotate out until you reach a 45 to 60-degree angle. (It is possible to go as far as a 90-degree angle if your hips are sufficiently flexible, but you must work up to this over time). When you reach the desired angle, pause. Then, slowly rotate back toward the right, moving through the starting position until your knee points 30 to 45 degrees to the right. Pause and then repeat.

You will feel your hip muscles contracting as they move through their external and internal rotation ranges of motion. As you progress with this exercise, you will reach the point where you are able to execute this movement without your hands on the wall.

## EXERCISES FOR STRENGTHENING/ENDURANCE

### *Hand-resisted Isometrics*

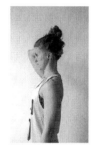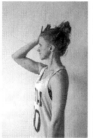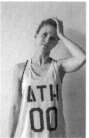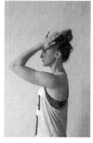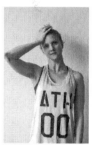

*Hand-resisted isometrics* are one of the lowest-level exercises you can perform to strengthen your neck.

To perform this exercise, begin by performing a chin tuck motion so that your head is in alignment with the rest of your body. From there, bring your hand up and place it directly against your forehead. Slowly apply some pressure with your hand and resist the movement with your neck muscles. This will strengthen the muscles on the front of your neck.

To exercise the rest of your neck muscles, one method is to place your right hand flat against the right side of your head and push into it. Alternatively, place your left hand flat against the left side of your head and push into it. Finally, another method is to place one hand on the back of your head and push forward.

### Chair Neck Tilts

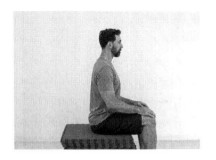 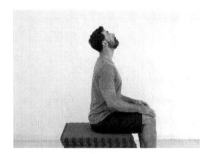

*Chair neck tilts* are an intermediate progression between standing flexion and extension, using the force of gravity on your head to add more resistance to your neck muscles. This allows you to slowly and progressively increase the resistance on your neck muscles through a range of motion without using any external weight.

You will start sitting upright in a chair. Allow your neck to slowly tilt back as you control the movement into extension. As you reach the end of the tilt, pause and slowly bring your neck back to the starting position, using the muscles in the front of your neck to complete the exercise.

This exercise can be progressed by moving your hips forward in the chair to increase the angle at which your neck leans. As you increase the angle over time, this will slowly make the exercise more and more difficult.

### Neck Flexion (Supine on Elbows)

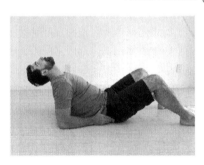 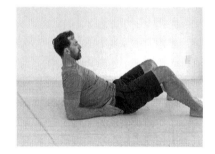

A good alternative to chair neck tilts is *neck flexion (supine on elbows)*.

Begin by laying on your back. Prop yourself up on your elbows so your body, arm, and forearm form a triangle. You may feel some stretching in the front of your shoulders and chest. This is normal and good. From this position, begin facing forward and slowly lower your head back until you reach the end of your range. Pause and then slowly return your head to the starting position.

Although this is an alternative to chair neck tilts, this exercise provides the front of your shoulders and chest an excellent stretching sensation that many people never feel. Those who complete this exercise will usually find themselves "more free" to move. This is why I prefer this exercise over chair neck tilts, provided that you are able to work your way up to it.

### *Quadruped Neck Extension / Neck Extension (Elbows Prone)*

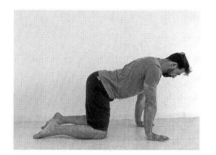 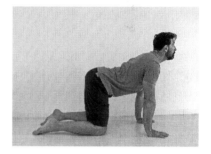

For the *quadruped neck extension*, begin on your hands and knees. Your shoulder and hip angles should be at 90 degrees. For the *neck extension (elbows prone)*, begin by resting your elbows on a soft, flat surface. Your back will naturally be arched and your stomach and legs should rest on the floor, a mattress, or other supportive surface.

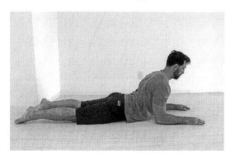 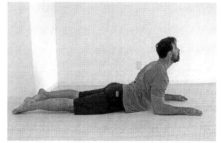

From each of these positions, begin by facing forward. Slowly lower your head until your chin touches your chest or your forehead touches the floor. Pause and slowly bring your head back up until you are looking forward.

These two positions mimic those that infants and toddlers go through while learning to move. Each of these positions demonstrate solid head control and allows the neck to strengthen itself in a normal movement pattern.

### Neck Flexion and Extension (Prone and Supine on Bed/Table)

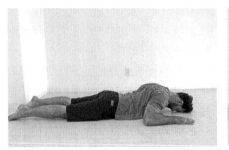 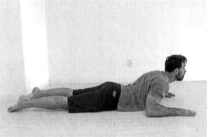

Prone and Supine Positions

You will begin this exercise by lying on your stomach on a bed or table. From there, slowly position yourself so that your whole body is still on the bed but your neck and head are off the bed. Relax your neck and slowly allow gravity to lower it down. Once you reach the bottom of the movement, use the muscles in the back of your neck to raise your neck up until you are looking straight ahead. Pause and slowly lower back down to the bottom of the movement once again.

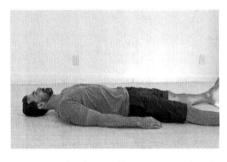 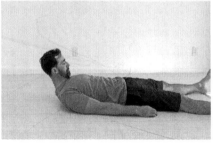

Begin by lying flat on your back. From there slowly bring your chin up toward your chest. Pause and slowly lower your head back to the ground.

Some people may experience dizziness, lightheadedness, or other symptoms during these movements. If this happens to you, stop exercising and consult a medical professional. If you only experience stretching sensations, that is acceptable.

This exercise is the last progression of the neck-strengthening and endurance exercises beginning from the upright position and ending lying down. These exercises all utilize the force of gravity on the head to strengthen the neck muscles. If you are working to increase neck strength beyond this, you may consider wrestler's bridges or neck harnesses. Of course, exercising your neck with added weight can be dangerous, so consult a medical professional before performing any of these movements.

### Face Pulls

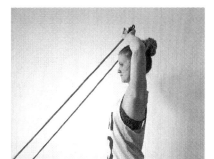

*Face pulls* are usually performed with a dumbbell or band. If you do not have this equipment, you can use objects around your home like soup cans, books, or a backpack filled with weight (and so on). If you do this, you will need to modify the exercise to allow gravity to work at a good angle. The most common way to do this is to perform a bent-over face pull.

There are a few different variations of this exercise. One is more like a row for the neck area. However, the variation that I prefer is the one that ends with a double biceps pose. This strengthens the muscles around your scapula and your shoulder external rotators at the same time.

For a regular face pull (with a machine or band), you will begin from a standing position. The first step is to grip the rope cable or band with both hands. Next, begin to pull back on the band or rope cable (like a row). However, you will not complete the rest of the movement like a row (where you pull until your hands reach your chest/armpits). Instead, make an upright "L" with your arms as you begin to pull back. Bring your arms back until they are in alignment with the rest of your body and can squeeze both of your scapula together. At the end position, your arms should be at shoulder height, straight out, and possessing a 90-degree bend at the elbow so that your forearms are sticking straight up. This is very similar to the basic position you use when you stretch your biceps.

### Band External Rotation with Retraction

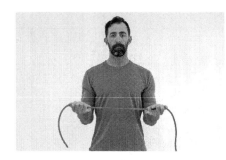 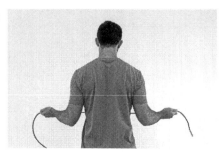

You can begin in a sitting or standing position with your arms by your side. First, bend your elbows to a 90-degree angle while stretching a band between them. Next, rotate both of your hands out to the side in order to bring them into alignment with the rest of your body. When you begin to bring your hands out to the side, you should also squeeze both of your scapulas together tightly. Do not allow your shoulders to "shrug" up to ear-level; rather, keep them down as far as possible.

This exercise is good for strengthening the scapular retraction muscles and the external rotators of the shoulders. These tend to be weak and/or underutilized in most populations, including the sedentary and many different types of athletes. This is also a good exercise for opening up the chest, which may get tight when one's shoulders round forward.

## Inverted Rows / Dumbell (DB) Rows

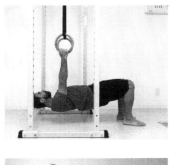 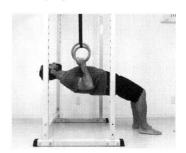

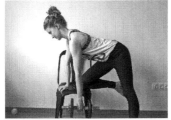 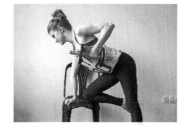

*Inverted rows* usually require equipment like rings or parallel bars, or a way to lower a bar in the gym, such as a Smith machine. For this exercise, grab the bar or rings with both hands. Next, position your body so that it is straight and squeeze your glutes, abdominals, and leg muscles. Make sure that your body does not sag down into a curve or bowl shape. From there, squeeze your scapulas back and pull your hands so that the rings or bar come to the bottom of your rib cage. Keep your elbows tucked during the movement. Pause at the top position where the rings or bar make contact with your body. Lower slowly back down to the starting position.

You can also progress with this exercise by moving your elbows out to form a 90-degree angle with your torso and bring the bar or rings to chest-height. This will modify the angle of the exercise on your back muscles, which helps emphasize the posterior part of your shoulder and scapular muscles more effectively.

For *dumbbell rows* (also called *DB rows*), there are many different useful variations you can utilize. The one I want to teach you today is the *one-arm dumbbell row*. This movement requires dumbbells and a bench so it can be performed easily in a gym setting or at home with a chair/couch and a dumbbell.

You will begin in a standing position. First, bend over while keeping one hand flat on the bench or raised surface. Keep your legs and back straight, hips bent at 90-degree angle, and arm angle at 90 degrees from your torso. Pick up the dumbbell and allow it to hang freely. Begin to pull with your elbow tucked in toward your body and retract your scapula. Continue to pull the weight up until it reaches your armpit area and touches your chest. Pause before slowly lowering to the starting position.

With this exercise, there is often a tendency to use momentum from the bottom of the movement, but you should resist the urge to do this. Perform the first set with your weak arm before switching to your other arm. You can progress in this exercise by using heavier weights.

### Hollow Hold and Superman Hold

The *hollow hold* and *superman hold* are basic body positioning holds that improve your level of body positioning endurance. For solid benefits, you can generally progress to the point where each hold can be performed for roughly 60 seconds.

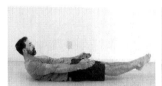 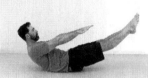 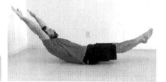

Hollow Hold

Begin by lying on your back with your arms next to your body. Slowly lift your legs off the ground, keeping them straight by contracting your abdominals. In the same manner, slowly lift your upper body off the ground by rounding your chest slightly. Your body should form a slight C shape and your lower back should be against the ground. If possible, only your lower back should touch the ground.

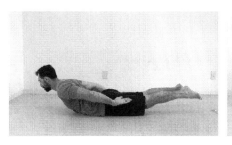 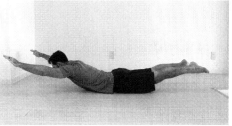

Superman Hold

Begin by lying on your stomach with your arms next to your body. Slowly lift your legs off the ground, keeping them straight by contracting your glutes and back muscles. In the same manner, slowly lift your upper body off the ground by arching your chest slightly. Your body should form a slight C shape and your stomach should be against the ground. If possible, only your stomach should touch the ground.

You can begin this exercise with your hands next to your body and progress by extending your arms overhead. You can also progress by adding a dynamic movement while maintaining the shape. To do this, rock forward and backward (like a seesaw) for each of the motions. These are called *hollow rocks* and *superman rocks*, respectively.

### Quadruped Kicks and Fire Hydrants

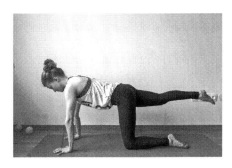 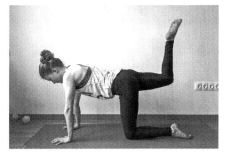

*Quadruped kicks* are also called *donkey kicks*, begin on your hands and knees. Your shoulder and hip angles should be at 90 degrees. Kick your right leg out behind you. At the same time, keep your 90-degree shoulder and hip angles the same and resist the urge to move your torso. This will help you isolate your glutes and hamstrings. Continue to kick your leg straight back until it is straight and in alignment with the rest of your body. Really squeeze your glutes when you perform this exercise! Repeat on the opposite side. These are great basic glute activation and endurance drills you can perform to get your glutes firing well!

One of the alternatives to this movement (which you may feel more effectively in your glutes) is to keep the knee of your kicking leg bent at a 90-degree angle for the entire duration of the movement.

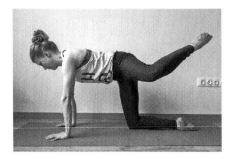 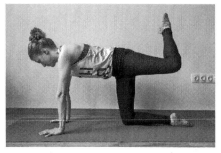

*Fire hydrants* are another glute exercise that focuses more on different heads of your gluteal muscles. It is named as such because it resembles the way male dogs pee on fire hydrants.

To perform this exercise, begin on your hands and knees. Your shoulder and hip angles should be 90 degrees. Keep your knee bent at a 90-degree angle and lift your right leg up to the side. Resist the urge to rotate your torso while you perform this movement. Once you reach the limit of your range of motion, pause and then slowly lower your leg back down. Repeat on the opposite side.

*Circular fire hydrants* are an excellent way to progress this exercise through a varied range of motion, and they are also beneficial for increased glute activation and endurance training. This exercise is the same as standard fire hydrants, but instead of lowering at the top of the movement you will keep your leg up and begin to rotate it back behind you. It should end in a similar position as the quadruped/donkey kicks and you can then lower back down to the ground.

This exercise can be performed in reverse order, beginning with the donkey kick and then moving to the fire hydrant position before lowering down. I recommend that you become comfortable with both variations.

Both quadruped kicks and fire hydrants are very basic glute activation and endurance drills that you can perform to get your glutes firing properly.

### Reverse Hyperextensions

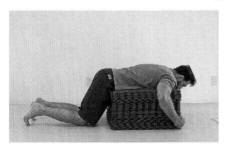 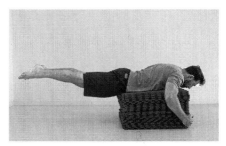

To perform a *reverse hyperextension*, you need to have a stable block, table, bed, or otherwise raised surface that you can lie on and hold onto. First, place your torso on the surface of your choice and secure yourself by gripping the edge of the object. (Alternatively, if there is nothing to grip, you can use a backpack filled with heavy books or a similar object to prevent yourself from rocking backward while performing the exercise.) Next, keep your legs straight and slowly use your glutes and back to raise your legs straight up behind you. Continue until your body forms a straight line. Pause before slowly lowering your lower body. Pause again at the bottom of the movement. Repeat as necessary.

One regression that can be made to this exercise is bending the knees. This modification shortens the lever of your legs, which makes the exercise easier to perform. As you progress, you can gradually bend your knees less while performing this exercise. Those who get fairly strong can also add ankle weights or other types of resistance in order to increase the level of difficulty.

Reverse hyperextensions are one of my favorite exercises to help athletes rehabilitate their backs. We have found that *back extensions*—a similar movement—do not work as effectively for rehabilitation. This is because back extensions are primarily a hip-hinge exercise, which keeps your torso straight for the duration of the movement. Reverse hyperextensions have the same hip-hinging technique, but the back acts as a stabilizer for your entire lower body. This is why we have seen better results with reverse hyperextensions than with back extensions in many cases.

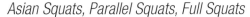

*Asian Squats, Parallel Squats, Full Squats*

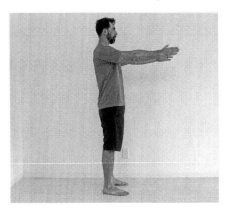
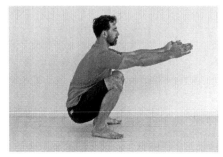

While children are able to easily move in and out of the squat position, many adults have difficultly comfortably moving into a squat. Therefore, the *Asian squat* is a great technique to train your body to become re-accustomed to the bottom position of a squat, particularly if you have been inactive for an extended period of time.

This position can be used to assess your mobility and overall flexibility. Learning to move in and out of a squat comfortably is not just beneficial for maintaining mobility and flexibility, but also for re-learning the foundations of human movement.

Keep your feet roughly shoulder width apart or slightly wider, with your toes turned out from zero to thirty degrees based on what is most comfortable for you. Initiate the movement like you are sitting back in a chair. Keep your weight over or slightly behind the middle of your foot. Descend until your thighs touch the backs of your calves, while keeping your back straight. Do not let your back round at the bottom of the movement. If you have good squat mobility, the backs of your thighs should touch your calves. From there, raise your body in the same manner that you descended. Keep your back straight and utilize the power through your hips and knees.

Those who spend a lot of time sitting may experience difficulty with this movement and compensate by allowing their knees to move excessively in front of their toes. Your knees should move over your toes to maintain correct alignment, but you should sit back enough to where you are using your hip muscles as well.

The primary difference between a *parallel squat* and the *full squat* is the range of motion. In the parallel squat, you descend until your thighs are parallel, whereas in the full squat you descend until your thighs touch the backs of your calves. The latter requires more mobility and flexibility, which can be difficult for those who are accustomed to sitting. If you observe any toddler, you will find that most can easily do a full squat, an ability that is often lost as we become adults and are less active. Our muscles thus become accustomed to shorter ranges, which limit our range of motion and make it difficult to perform many exercises like squats.

If you need to begin with a parallel squat, that is perfectly fine. Likewise, if your heels come off the floor when you start, you may place a small piece of wood or other material under your heels so you can achieve good depth during the squat. Stretch your hamstrings and calves so that you can eventually remove the heel-lift.

Some people have difficulty keeping their knees tracking over the toes. One of the most common faults with the squat is that your knees may collapse toward one another. This fault can place a lot of stress on your ACL, MCL, and meniscus. In sports, when an athlete injures all three of these muscles at once, it is called an "unhappy triad." Thus, it is imperative to learn how to keep your knees tracking correctly. If you have trouble getting a feel for this, you can place a TheraBand or other stretchy material around your knees. This will cue you to keep your knees out while you perform a squat.

### Side-to-side Squats / Cossack Squats

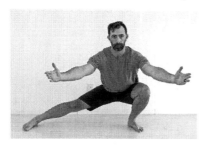 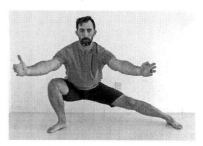

The *side-to-side squat* is also known as a *Cossack squat*. It is useful as a precursor for lunges, deep step-ups, and pistols because it biases your weight onto either leg as you move from side to side.

Begin in a standing straddle position. Slowly shift your weight to your left (or right) and slowly lower your body until your butt touches your calf on one side. Next, stand up through the movement until your legs are straight and then slowly lower to the other side. Repeat for your desired number of repetitions.

If this exercise is too difficult to perform from a full squat position, elevate your feet with a mat or other implement in order to make it easier to bend. Alternatively, you can hold onto a door or sturdy table in order to assist the bottom portion of the movement.

The goal is to eventually go down to the thigh-to-calf or butt-to-calf range for this exercise. The toes of your straight leg can point forward if you want to stretch your adductors, or upward if you want to stretch your hamstrings more. Make sure you use your leg strength to push out of the bottom of the movement and move slowly in order to improve mobility/flexibility. If you would like to stretch your hips further, simply rest momentarily in the bottom of the movement.

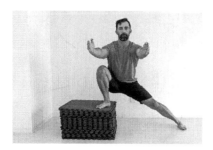 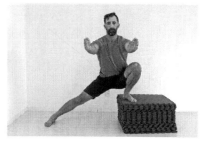

If you find it difficult to perform a full squat with this exercise, you can elevate your feet with a mat or other implement. Alternatively, you can hold onto a door or sturdy table for assistance in the bottom portion of the movement.

### Foot Drills

*Foot drills* are one of the best exercises for rehabilitation after ankle sprains. These drills are used widely for track and field athletes and I know several coaches who utilize them with their athletes. Foot drills are also good for sedentary individuals and athletes who do not have sprains because they teach good proprioception and kinesthetic awareness for the feet. This is important because we often stand, walk, or run a certain way, and these exercises strengthen the muscles in positions that we do not often find ourselves in naturally. This means if you ever "take a wrong step," your body has been trained in a way that should help mitigate injuries.

Additionally, strengthening your feet and regaining range of motion at your ankles (in conjunction with the hip-strengthening and range-of-motion exercises) helps take stress off your knees and promote healthy knee function.

There are six different foot drills. For each of these, you will walk 25 to 50 feet forward, turn around, and walk back.

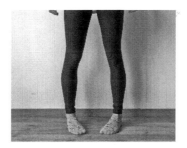

**Feet Pointed In** — Turn your feet in so they point toward each other. The angle can vary depending on your range of motion; anywhere from 30 to 45 degrees is good. (If you cannot turn your feet in that far, work on improving your inner hip range of motion.) Slowly walk forward while keeping your feet in this position. As you are walking, you may feel inactive muscles in your feet and hips begin to fire.

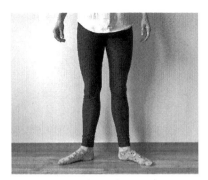

**Feet Pointed Out** — Turn your feet out so they point away from each other. The angle can vary depending on your range of motion; anywhere from 30 to 45 degrees is good. (If you cannot turn your feet in that far, work on improving your outer hip range of motion.) Slowly walk forward while keeping your feet in this position. As you are walking, you may feel inactive muscles in your feet and hips begin to fire.

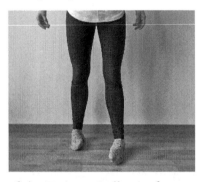

**On the Outside of the Foot** — Roll your foot out slightly, so that only the outside of your foot is touching the ground while the inside of your foot is slightly off the ground. (Do not roll your foot so far out that your ankle rolls over and you sprain it.) Next, slowly walk forward while keeping your feet positioned in this manner. As you are walking, you may feel the muscles in your feet and the inside of your legs begin to fire.

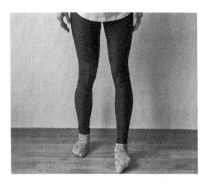

**On the Inside of the Foot** — Roll your foot in slightly, so that only the inside of your foot is touching the ground while the outside of your foot is slightly off the ground. Slowly walk forward while keeping your feet positioned in this manner. As you are walking, you may feel the muscles in your feet and the outside of your legs begin to fire.

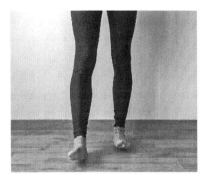

**Walking on Your Heels** — Slowly lift the front of your foot off the ground, so that only the heels of both of your feet are in contact with the ground. It may be difficult to maintain your balance while doing this. Slowly walk forward while keeping your feet positioned in this manner. As you are walking, you may feel the muscles in the front of your legs begin to fire.

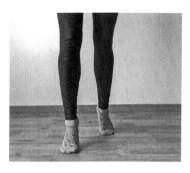

**Walking Backward on Your Toes with Your Heels Off the Ground** — Slowly raise your heels off of the ground so that you are only standing on the front of your feet or "tippie toes." It may be difficult to maintain your balance while doing this. Slowly walk backward while keeping your feet positioned in this manner. As you are walking, you may feel the muscles in the back of your legs begin to fire.

You may notice that it is more difficult to perform these drills with your feet pointed in than it is to perform them with your feet pointed out. You may also notice that walking on the insides of your feet is more difficult than walking on the outsides of your feet. Both of these scenarios are normal.

Most people's feet are turned out to some degree and are prone to inversion sprains where their foot rolls inward. This can be prevented by practicing more difficult variations of foot drills. You can also work the rest of your muscles near your ankle and leg by walking backward on your heels and the tips of your toes.

## OTHER EXERCISES

There are certainly more exercises that could have been included in this book, many of which may be very effective for you. In *Overcoming Gravity*, I (Steven) included hundreds of exercises; however, I understand that most of us have busy schedules and thus only have time for short exercise sessions. Therefore, I have attempted to provide the most "bang for your buck" with the exercises I have included in *Overcoming Poor Posture*. These are the exercises I feel will help you the most, but you may come across others that are just as effective or perhaps more so.

The exercises I have suggested for improving mobility, stability, flexibility, and endurance, and strength are not meant to replace an existing workout routine in your training regimen. They may become part of your training, but they are in no way a substitute for resistance training or cardiovascular exercise and may not help you reach your other goals related to health, athletic performance, aesthetics, and so on. You should also note that adding these exercises to your routine may help improve your overall performance, as improvement in one area (in this case, better movement) can bleed over into other areas.

Other systems of movement like yoga or Pilates, which emphasize control and mastery of movement and positions, may also be effective. Feel free to take the suggestions in this chapter and add to or subtract from them in order to construct a routine that works for you (something you can do with any program). However, be mindful of the fact that deviation from a program may result in different results than what the program was designed to help you attain. This may not be an issue with this topic, as being able to move effectively is generally good for numerous areas of training.

As you learn to move more effectively, remember to begin with basic isolation exercises. As you progress, you can move to more complex and difficult movements.

In general, we learn as infants to move effectively through crawling, rolling, squatting, and other basic movements that are foundational to human development. Many physical therapy and rehabilitation exercises resemble these movements because they are able to retrain your nervous system to move effectively once again. When in doubt, go back to the basics.

### Resets

Generally speaking, *postural resets* are not really "resets" in the sense that they will fix your posture. Instead, they are positions that emphasize or overemphasize positions that are rarely attained in everyday work and life. Thus, they can help minimize the discomfort of being in certain problematic postural positions. You will find that if and when you use postural resets, it is much easier to move freely.

*Hyperextension Pose*

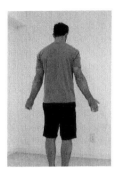 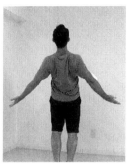 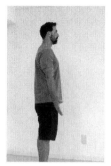 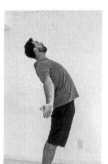

This movement involves spinal hyperextension, scapular depression and retraction, and arm external rotation. Here are the steps you will take to achieve it:

1. First, stand up straight with a proud chest.

2. Bring your arms out to your side, with your palms facing forward to form an arrow (with your head at the top). Your arms and torso should create a 45-degree angle.

3. Next, externally rotate your shoulders as far as possible so that your thumbs are now pointing sideways. You will eventually want them to point backward if possible.

4. Retract and depress your scapulas as far as you are able.

5. Follow up the aforementioned movement by arching your back slowly. Stop before you move into a range that causes you to feel any discomfort. This will open up your thoracic spine and create a nice stretching sensation in your chest and abdominal region.

6. Hold this position. Perform some deep breathing exercises, relaxing your muscles as you exhale and contracting them as you inhale. Try breathing in, holding your breath for a few seconds, and then slowly exhaling through pursed lips. As you exhale, relax your traps and allow your shoulders to sink further back until they are retracted and depressed.

After you finish this exercise and relax for a bit, you should be able to sit or stand without much, if any, discomfort in your posture. It should not be long before you notice you are able to move much more effectively.

### Wall Fix/Band Fix

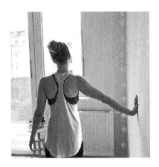 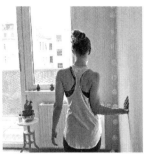 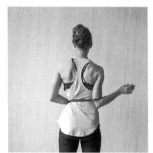

This forced scapular retraction and spinal extension exercise works great for easing pain, discomfort, or tension around your shoulder blades. In my experience, it is very effective for those involved in gymnastics, parkour, climbing, and even for Olympic lifters training the overhead position.

There are two setups that you can use for this exercise:

- You can use a TheraBand to forcibly retract your scapula(s), as shown in the above image.
- Alternatively, you can face parallel to the wall, place your hand against the wall and extend your arm outward. Step toward the wall while keeping your elbow behind your body in order to force your scapula into retraction.

Once you have used one of the above methods to get into position, you will complete three simple steps to help encourage better posture, release stress, open up your chest area, and decrease the amount of tension on your back muscles. All of these, when performed together, will cause you to experience less pain, discomfort, and/or tension in your neck and scapular area.

1. Begin with deep breathing. Inhale through your nose for four seconds and then exhale slowly through your mouth for eight seconds. If you desire, you can hold your breath for five seconds and puff up your chest to generate tension in the surrounding muscles.

The goal is to build tension by contracting your muscles, and to release this tension as you exhale. This should begin to loosen up the anterior portion of your shoulder.

2.  Work on scapular retraction holds. With your shoulder blades forcibly retracted, contract your muscles to pull your shoulder blades as close to your spine as possible. Hold this position for ten seconds. Repeat three to five times for each shoulder blade. This will release any tension and help orient your muscles to an optimal posture.

3.  Finally, squeeze your shoulder blades together once again. Slowly shrug up and down to maximal shoulder blade elevation and depression. Your range of motion should be between four to six inches as you move your shoulder blades up toward your ears and back down toward your lower back. Pause for three to five seconds at the top and bottom portions of this movement in order to contract your muscles, which will happen naturally.

After completing these three steps, evaluate your posture. These movements should open up your chest area and decrease muscle tightness in the front of your shoulders. They should also relieve discomfort and tension from the back of your shoulder blades, which is particularly beneficial if you carry tension or stress in your shoulders. In the vast majority of cases, you will feel much better when you stand up straight as well.

These movements over-exaggerate proper alignment in order to move you into a more neutral range upon completion. Deep breathing helps relax your muscles and release tension, and the retractions with elevation and depression eliminate tension and reorient your muscles to their proper resting lengths.

*Chair/Parallettes/Box Fix*

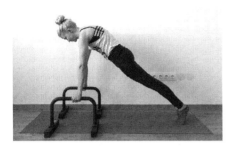 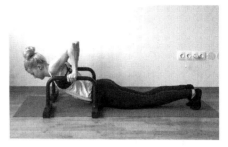

This postural reset is a forced scapular retraction and spinal extension. Here are the steps you will take to perform it:

1. Get two chairs or stools that are about knee height. Alternatively, you can use a set of parallettes or a box.
2. Begin in a pushup position, with your hands on the raised implements of your choice. Slowly lower into the bottom of the pushup position.
3. Relax and allow the force of gravity to drag your elbows backward and force your scapulas to retract and stretch out your chest.
4. Allow your back to arch into thoracic extension within a comfortable range. Hold this position while breathing deeply for thiry seconds.

Your lower body does not have any "highly effective positions" that can loosen up everything, like your upper body does. However, a sequence of movements can be particularly effective.

One particular sequence that I have found works well involves moving through:

- Hip Flexor Stretching
- Regular Squatting
- Cossack Squats
- Foot Drills

If your lifestyle involves a lot of prolonged sitting, adding quadruped kicks and/or fire hydrants right after the hip flexor stretch may work well for you.

- Hip Flexor Stretching
- Quadruped Kicks and/or Fire Hydrants
- Regular Squatting
- Cossack Squats
- Foot Drills

The sequence above may not negate the effects of long-term sitting, but it should help mitigate the most detrimental effects. One of the important elements of hip health is simply getting your hips moving. The cartilage in your hip socket is avascular, which means it does not receive a blood supply at all but instead receives nutrients from the movement of your hip joints, which stimulate the flow of synovial fluid within your hip socket.

## CHAPTER SUMMARY

o   The corrective exercises presented in this chapter are grouped into the following categories:

- *Mobility* and *Stability*, which improve your range of motion and control, both dynamically and statically.

- *Strength* and *Endurance*, which improve your ability to maintain and move into proper postural alignments.

- *Resets*, which are exaggerated positions that help improve your body awareness for attaining better positioning.

## FURTHER STUDY

- North American Journal of Sports Physical Therapy article on segmental rolling in athletes for an increase in control and coordination: www.ncbi.nlm.nih.gov/pmc/articles/PMC2953329

- International Journal of Sports Physical Therapy article on segmental rolling in athletes for an increase in control and coordination: www.ncbi.nlm.nih.gov/pmc/articles/PMC4637914

## Chapter 7

# CHANGING YOUR HABITS

S o far, we have offered many useful exercises and strategies that will help develop your physical structure. However, it is important to understand that your everyday habits have an equal effect on your posture. The way you hold your body and your default positions while sitting and standing are the result of years of conditioning, whether good or bad. These habits can be difficult to change.

Just as in the familiar example of people getting excited and gung ho about their New Year's resolutions, only to burn out a few weeks later, working on improving your posture can follow the same route if you aren't careful.

Changing your habits is a discipline in itself and can easily require a specific program. In this chapter, we will attempt to provide the most important information related to forming habits that will change your posture. Executing these strategies will help you get the most out of this book and stay consistent with your goals to improve your posture.

## PRACTICAL APPLICATIONS OF HABIT CHANGE

### Avoid Extremes

Avoid the trap of perfectionism in every facet of your postural correction plan. Avoid extremes, such as devising a daily postural exercise plan that takes two hours to complete, setting a timer to check your posture every five minutes, or using tape, a harness, or any other postural aid to keep your shoulders back. These other techniques may sound good, but you will quickly burn out. Postural correction takes time to achieve, and the results are difficult to see on a daily basis. Therefore, it is much better to take consistent "good" steps than inconsistent "perfect steps."

> "Perfect is the enemy of the good."

In *Overcoming Poor Posture*, we lay out many types of exercises and strategies you can utilize, but there is no need to implement all of them at the same time. We have attempted to offer a wide variety of suggestions so you can find what works for you, rather than prescribing a set plan that must be followed without deviation.

We recommend starting with much *less* than you think you can accomplish. Remember, the secret is *consistency*, not *quantity*. We recommend being consistent with a few exercises for at least two weeks before adding more. It is better to add more later than to begin with more and have to subtract because, frankly, most people don't just subtract, they stop completely.

## Motivation

There are two primary types of motivation in psychological theory: *intrinsic* and *extrinsic*. Intrinsic motivation is defined as an enjoyment of the activity itself, whereas extrinsic motivations are a desire for a reward or a prize.

It is too simple to value one form of motivation over the other, such as saying it is much better to enjoy the process than to pursue the benefits. Both contribute to goal-setting and habit-change depending on various factors such as: an individual's personality, the type of reward/prize, how often a reward is given, and so on.

You'll have to do a bit of soul-searching and analyze your past history to see what is best for you. Are you the type of person that enjoys simply doing an exercise program or other regimen? If so, you won't need some kind of reward. In fact, research has shown that if you have good intrinsic motivation, the addition of extrinsic rewards decreases interest in the activity.

On the other hand, do you realize that you need some type of reward to be consistent with something? Whether the milestone is time ("Once I exercise every day for two weeks straight") or achievement ("once I can easily do three sets of twelve on this exercise"), you can treat yourself to a reward ("I'll give myself X.").

There is a relationship between both types of motivation. Over time, the intrinsic enjoyment of an activity increases as the benefits accrue. It goes without saying, but you tend to enjoy something more when it brings you rewards.[24]

An honest assessment of your attitude toward a regimen will play a huge role in your success.

## Neuroplasticity

*Neuroplasticity* has been a bit of a buzzword for the past few years. In particular, Norman Doidge's *The Brain That Changes Itself* is a popular science book that made the term widely known. Simply put, neuroplasticity means that what was once thought to be immutable and fixed can be changed with practice and effort.

Just knowing this can be profound. Habit change requires breaking associations and replacing past perceptions with new realities. To achieve that, you must have a firm belief that you can actually change.

It seems silly to even state that, because surely everyone who picks up a book like this or does any kind of exercise program must believe that they can change themselves. But these self-doubts can creep up on you, and with the low rate of adherence to regular exercise, it's essential to have a solid foundation of *self-efficacy* (one's belief in one's ability to succeed in specific situations or accomplish a task).[25]

Physical transformations (losing weight, gaining muscle) and habitual pattern changes require consistent effort, time, and patience. Every bit of the process can be challenging. It's difficult to begin a program, to press on during inevitable plateaus, and even difficult to maintain once certain goals are achieved. Therefore, it is imperative to have an adaptable and flexible mindset in order to stay on course.

> "Plant a thought and reap a word;
> plant a word and reap an action;
> plant an action and reap a habit;
> plant a habit and reap a character;
> plant a character and reap a destiny."

"Plant a thought and reap a word; plant a word and reap an action; plant an action and reap a habit; plant a habit and reap a character; plant a character and reap a destiny."

While this quote has been attributed to many people, the thought is profound. Even though you may not be attempting to transform your character or destiny, you are trying to develop good habits. This is why it is important to follow through on your thoughts, words, and actions; it is how good habits are formed, and these habits will help shape your body's athletic ability and overall health for the long haul.

## STEPS TO TAKE RIGHT NOW

### Identify Your Motivation for Change

- What is your primary reason for wanting to change your posture?

- What will keep you motivated and consistent in your plan to improve?

- Schedule checkpoints on a weekly basis to reassess whether your motives and plans are still the most relevant for you. Change and adapt as necessary!

### Organize Your Plan

- Pick one of the sample plans we provide that appeals the most to you based on how much time and energy you have in your schedule. Consider cutting that plan in half in terms of number of exercises and the recommendations for sets and reps. Start there and build over time. It's better to start small and keep going than to swing for the fences and give up when frustration hits.

- Build your own plan from the strategies we share, individualizing them to fit your schedule and personal needs. As mentioned above, be conservative and begin with less of everything so you can build a consistent habit first. Don't overdo it at the start and end up stopping early!

- Schedule checkpoints every two weeks to reassess your plan. Consider how consistent you've been, what exercises and strategies worked well, and what continues to be challenging for you.

## CHAPTER SUMMARY

o   Habit change is essential for improving and maintaining physical changes.

o   Understanding the two types of motivation (intrinsic and extrinsic) can help you persist in your training and avoid dropping out. Do you need to work toward a reward, or is the training itself motivation enough? We tend to cycle through both at different points in our lives.

o   Neuroplasticity refers to the nervous system's ability to change through repetition and adaptation. We are what we practice, and over time, we can change what was once thought to be static and unchangeable.

o   Implement habit and mindset practice in your physical training plan immediately to accrue the most benefits from your efforts.

## FURTHER STUDY

- *The Brain That Changes Itself*, book by Norman Doidge, M.D. (New York: Penguin, 2007); available on Amazon.com.

## Chapter 8

# PROGRAMMING TO OVERCOME POOR POSTURE

## PURPOSE OF EXERCISES

The purpose of an exercise is important. One of the concepts often left unaddressed is how to maintain a new range of motion once you have obtained it. Generally, you should expect increases in range of motion if you are foam rolling, massaging, or performing joint mobilization or flexibility work. This, of course, does not always happen. Sometimes, particular muscles or joints tighten back up. While the previously mentioned issues of instability, weakness, or pain may prevent one from decreasing tight musculature, there could be another culprit.

Flexibility and mobility are similar, but not interchangeable. *Flexibility* is about increasing range of motion or muscle length by stretching. It is difficult to move a joint when the muscles surrounding that joint are not able to stretch. If you cannot touch your toes, performing flexibility work will elongate your hamstring muscles until you can.

On the other hand, *mobility* is an umbrella term that covers any movement within an existing range of motion. Typically, it is performed at lower intensities with just your bodyweight. Mobility has three specific goals: maintaining existing ranges of motion, improving motor learning, and increasing movement quality. If movement within an existing range of motion is loaded with weight or resistance at a high enough percentage of your one-repetition maximum, it will become strength or hypertrophy work.

Whenever you obtain a new range of motion, you should follow up by performing both passive and active mobility work in the new range. For example, if you stretched your ankle, you will want to follow up with passive mobility work that consists of moving your ankle in the new range manually, then actively contracting your muscles in the new range. This helps solidify your gains by providing feedback to your body that the new range of motion is safe and can be used effectively. Once this happens, your body will no longer send mechanoreceptor (pressure/distortion) or nociceptor (pain) feedback to your nervous system that causes your muscle spindles to sensitize and limit your range of motion.

Habits are hard to break. If your body has not been flexible for many years, it tends to revert to what it knows. Your muscle spindles may start to naturally sensitize even if you have not stretched into pain. This can happen very easily if you do not perform mobility or range-of-motion work.

The same is true in changing your posture. If you have had poor alignment for years, moving into a different alignment is going to be uncomfortable for a few weeks as your body adjusts to the new positioning. If you are seeking to make your body flexible for the first time in your life, you must get in the habit of stretching and performing mobility work on a daily basis, or even multiple times a day. This may be difficult at first, but once the new habit is established, you will be able to maintain your gains much more easily.

If you do nothing to maintain your range of motion, your body will tighten back up. This is why mobility and flexibility work outside of a workout routine is so important. Most people who are flexible and mobile are training these every day, not just on workout days. If you perform mobility work daily and flexibility work every other day, you should be able to maintain your range of motion gains. However, if you want to progress to the next range of motion quicker, performing both mobility and flexibility work on a daily basis is recommended. The phrase "use it or lose it!" applies to the SAID principle—specific adaptation to imposed demand. If you do not use your new range of motion, you will likely lose it before your next workout.

It is important to construct your workout routine with all your goals in mind, not just the workout itself. A routine designed to increase flexibility may only have you stretching a couple times a week; however, you really need to be performing mobility and flexibility work daily to reach your goal of becoming more flexible.

This frequency may seem unmanageable, but there are many ways to make mobility and flexibility a part of your daily routine, even if you keep a busy schedule. You can perform a little when you wake up and before you go to bed at night, or as you are preparing a meal. Whether or not you perform both mobility and flexibility daily depends on your goals, but the bottom line is that you need to do something every day.

Some people will be able to progress in flexibility while only stretching three times per week. Others may need to stretch multiple times per day, seven days per week. Then there are those who may need to stretch three to five times per week in addition to performing mobility work multiple times per day. If you notice your routine is not working, vary it to figure out what works best for you! Additionally, you can try adding PNF (Proprioceptive Neuromuscular Facilitation) or LS (Loaded Stretching) in your flexibility workouts.

## ORDERING OF EXERCISES

There is a method to the madness of ordering exercises in your workout. This order should pay particular attention to both progression and purpose. Typically, an order of exercises is constructed in this manner:

1. Any Massage and Soft Tissue Work and/or Heat
2. Light Stretching, Mobility, and Stability Work
3. Strength and Endurance Exercises
4. Mobility Work

The reasoning behind this structure is very simple:

- Soft Tissue Work and/or Heat: Generally speaking, loosening up painful and tightened muscles tends to help you move better. This is the correct application of soft tissue work (as you may recall from earlier). It does not fix the overarching problem, but it helps with the immediate need.

- Light Stretching, Mobility, and Stability Work: After soft tissue work, light stretching, mobility, and stability work can help calm your nervous system and effectively utilize your new range(s) of motion. This is necessary for your body to move comfortably in the ranges of motion that *should* feel normal but often do not. Stretching aims to gain new ranges of motion, mobility work seeks to utilize said ranges of motion, and stability work helps to solidify your new ranges of motion. Stretching alone may not solidify your range of motion gains because your body is not actively utilizing these ranges of motion. "Use it or lose it!" is one popular phrase that applies to new ranges of motion.

- Strength and Endurance Exercises: The previous movements help to warm up an area for specific attribute training, especially if there was prior weakness or a new range of motion has been recently attained. Generally speaking, you never want to train strength or endurance on dysfunction; thus, the first two phases in the order of exercises are present to ensure quality movements occur with good technique.

- Mobility Work and/or Stability Work: Finally, if needed, you will want to finish with additional mobility and stability work. This helps solidify any movement and range of motion you may have acquired during your exercise session. This does not always have to occur after strength and endurance work; it can also be performed throughout the day so new ranges of motion or movements do not become stiff and more difficult for you to obtain in the future.

This is the general structure for creating your own plan for overcoming poor posture. Everything you need has been outlined above, but discovering what works best for you is a process of trial and error.

In the appendix of this book, you will find sample plans that will help you reach a variety of goals. These can easily be added into your current training regimen.

## CHAPTER SUMMARY

o  Every exercise you perform should have a specific purpose, whether that is improving your range of motion, strength, or body awareness.

o  When you know the purpose of each exercise, you can more effectively select exercises for your program based on your individual needs.

o  Together, mobility and flexibility work help you gain and maintain new ranges of motion. Both need to be trained regularly in order to affect change.

o  The ideal frequency and intensity of exercise can be different for different individuals. Discovering what works best for you is a process of trial and error. We recommend beginning with lower frequency and intensity, and increasing from there if you are not progressing.

o  You will achieve optimal benefits when you order your postural training exercises correctly: soft tissue work and/or heat, light stretching, mobility, and stability work, strength and endurance work, and mobility/stability training to conclude your workout.

## FURTHER STUDY

• There are comprehensive sections that cover program design in the second edition of Steven Low's best-selling book, *Overcoming Gravity: A Systematic Approach to Gymnastics and Bodyweight Strength* (Houston: Battle Ground Creative, 2016); available on Amazon.com. More information on stevenlow.org.

- *NSCA's Guide to Program Design*, book from the National Strength and Conditioning Association (Champaign, IL: Human Kinetics, 2012); available on Amazon: www.amazon.com/Program -Design-Science-Strength-Conditioning/dp/0736084029

- International Journal of Sports Physical Therapy article that lays out an exercise program designed for injured athletes: www.ncbi.nlm .nih.gov/pmc/articles/PMC3164002

## Chapter 9

# CONCLUSION

Throughout this book, we've outlined how improving your posture can benefit you beyond simply "standing taller." Postural work can enhance your psychological outlook, improve your performance in physical activities, and help you assess and address your physical restrictions and weaknesses.

It's not just the endpoint of your postural goals that provides these benefits; it's also the practice of the plan itself. The process of changing your habits and the introspection that comes with it will give you much insight into how you are wired and your ability to work toward your goals for self-improvement, which will carry over into every area of your life.

The strategies and plans in this book can offer immediate gains, especially improved comfort while sitting for an extended period of time. Other benefits, however—such as visual improvements in posture and physical performance—can take longer to achieve. It's best to realize this sooner rather than later so you can find the best way for you to be consistent with your exercise routine.

This quote from Josh Hillis is applicable to so many aspects of personal change and self-improvement: "People totally overestimate what they can do in a month or three months, but they totally underestimate what they can do in a year."

Find what will keep you going for the next year or more and you'll be amazed at the changes that you will see take place in your life.

# APPENDIX

## EXERCISE LIST

*Chin Tucks*

- Supine
- Standing
- With Sidebending
- With Rotation
- 45-degree

*Hand-Resisted Isometrics*

- Flexion
- Extension
- Sidebending

*Chair Neck Tilts*

*Supine on Elbows Neck Flexion*

*Quadruped Neck Extension*

*Prone on Elbows Neck Extension*

*Prone Neck Extension*

*Supine Neck Flexion*

*Face Pulls*

*Band External Rotation with Retraction*

*Inverted Rows*

*One-Arm Dumbbell Rows*

*Supine Hooklying Anterior and Posterior Pelvic Tilt*

- Regular Version
- Sidebending Version

*Quadruped Cat/Camel*

*Quadruped Spinal Circles*

*Quadruped Spinal Sidebending (Wag Tail)*

*Elbows on Wall Thoracic Extension*

*Prone Extension Press*

*Segmental Rolling*

1. Facing Up, Right Arm Roll
2. Facing Down, Right Arm Roll
3. Facing Up, Left Arm Roll
4. Facing Down, Left Arm Roll
5. Facing Up, Right Leg Roll
6. Facing Down, Right Leg Roll
7. Facing Up, Left Leg Roll
8. Facing Down, Left Leg Roll

*Couch/Wall Hip Flexor Stretch*

*Standing Hand-Resisted Hip Flexion*

*Standing Hand-Resisted Hip Flexion Rotations*

*Hollow Body Hold*

*Superman Hold*

*Quadruped Kicks*

- Straight Knee
- Bent Knee

*Fire Hydrant*

- Regular
- Circular

*Reverse Hyperextension* .

*Squat*

*Side-to-Side (Cossack) Squat*

- Regular
- Elevated

*Walking Foot Drills*

- Feet Pointed In
- Feet Pointed Out
- On the Outside of the Foot
- On the Inside of the Foot
- Walking on the Heels
- Walking Backward on the Toes with the Heels Off the Ground

*Hyperextension Pose*

*Wall/Band Fix*

*Chair/Parallettes/Box Fix*

# SAMPLE PLANS

The following plans can fit easily into daily routines and were designed to apply to common situations and goals. Feel free to use them as examples for creating your own plan that suits your individual needs.

## BARE MINIMUM (FOR THOSE SHORT ON TIME)

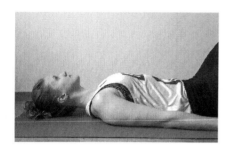 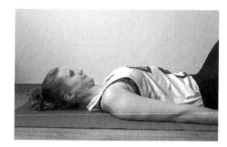

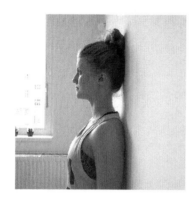 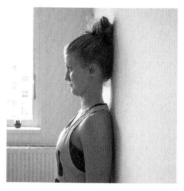

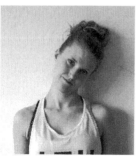 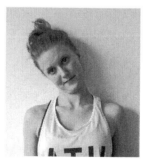

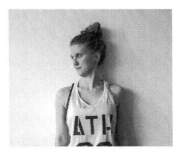

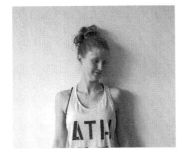

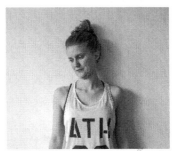

*Chin Tucks (Appropriate Variation) – Two Sets of Ten Repetitions*

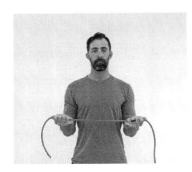

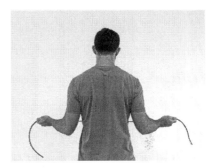

*Band External Rotation with Retraction – Two Sets of Twelve Repetitions*

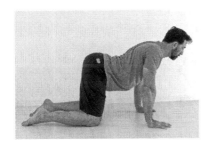

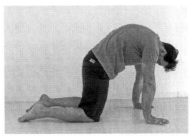

*Quadruped Cat/Camel – One Set of Ten Repetitions*

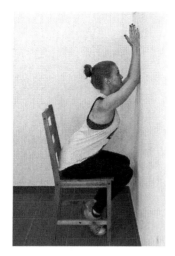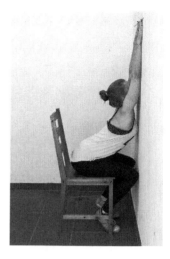

*Thoracic Extension (Elbows on Wall) – Two Sets of Thirty Seconds*

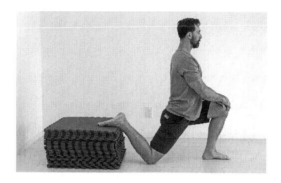

*Hip Flexor Stretch (Coach/Wall) – Two Sets of Thirty Seconds*

This plan is very efficient and emphasizes the primary areas that most people need to address in order to improve their posture.

You will begin with chin tucks, which address the very common head-forward posture. Choose the variation that is best for you. If you feel this exercise is too easy, begin with supine chin tucks. If this is still too easy, you may progress to the next variation.

To work on strength and mobility for your scapular and upper back muscles (which are often weak from lack of use during prolonged sitting, desk work, and/or driving) you will perform band external rotations with retractions.

To work on your spinal mobility and awareness (a necessary component of postural change), you will perform quadruped cat/camels and wall thoracic extension work.

Finally, the couch/wall hip flexor stretch will help loosen the muscles that affect your lower spine and pelvic positioning.

These five exercises will give you the most bang for your buck in terms of time investment.

## TRAINING WARM-UP/COOL DOWN

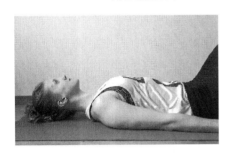 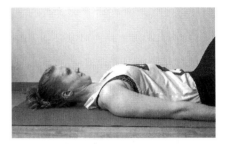

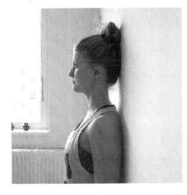 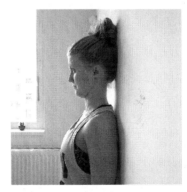

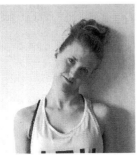 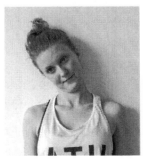

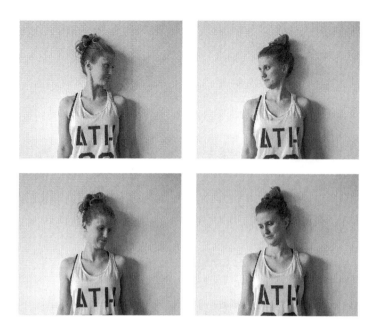

*Chin Tucks (Appropriate Variation) – Two Sets of Ten Repetitions*

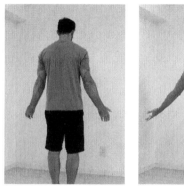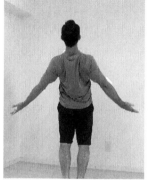

*Hyperextension Pose – Two Sets of Ten Repetitions*

## *Segmental Rolling – Three Repetitions of Each Roll*

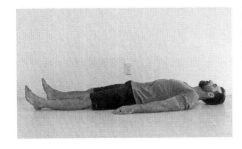
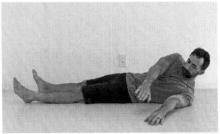

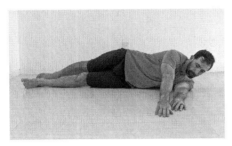
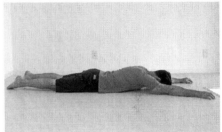

*Facing Up, Right Arm Roll*

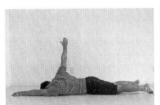
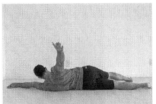
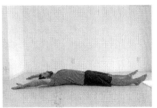

*Facing Down, Right Arm Roll*

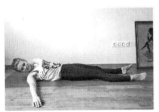
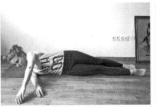
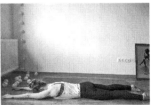

*Facing Up, Left Arm Roll*

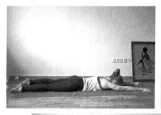
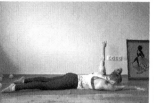
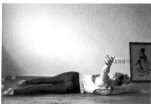
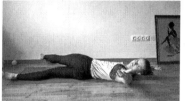
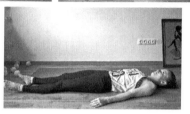

*Facing Down, Left Arm Roll*

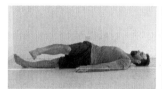
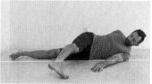
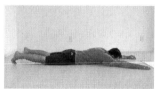

*Facing Up, Right Leg Roll*

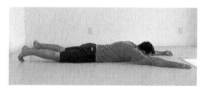
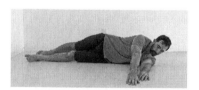
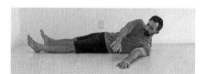
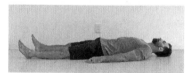

*Facing Down, Right Leg Roll*

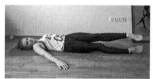
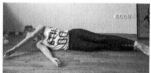
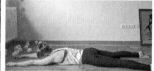

*Facing Up, Left Leg Roll*

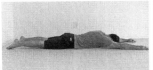 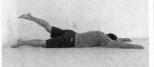 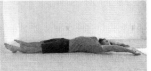

*Facing Down, Left Leg Roll*

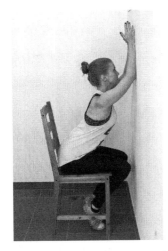 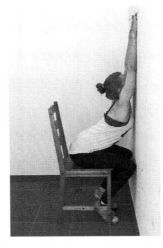

*Thoracic Extension (Elbows on Wall) – Three Sets of Thirty Seconds*

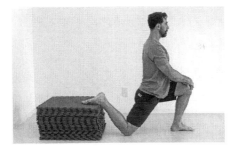

*Couch/Wall Hip Flexor Stretch – Three Sets of Thirty Seconds*

This series of exercises serves as a nice warm-up and cool down for your regular training sessions, with a blend of mobility and reset movements.

Choose one of the chin tuck exercise variations that works best for you. Begin with supine chin tucks and progress to the next variation if you feel they are too easy.

The hyperextension pose helps you "set" your posture, which will assist you in attaining good form for your training exercises (overhead presses, squats, etc.).

Segmental rolling is great for body awareness, muscle "timing," and coordination, which will help with your more dynamic exercises.

Wall thoracic extension work and the couch/wall hip flexor stretch target the more commonly stiff areas that most individuals have. Loosening these areas provides great benefits, both before and after training.

## ON THE JOB

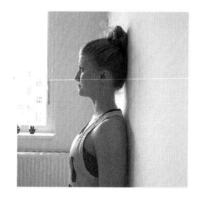 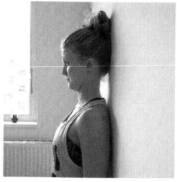

*Standing Chin Tucks (Appropriate Variation) – One Set of Ten Repetitions*

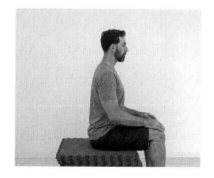 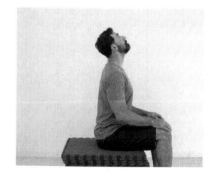

*Chair Neck Tilts – One Set of Ten Repetitions*

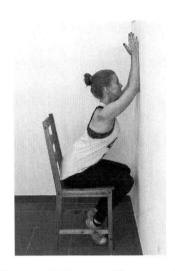 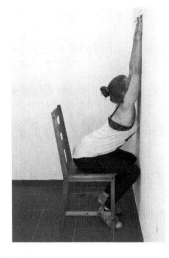

*Thoracic Extension (Elbows on Wall) – One Set of Thirty Seconds*

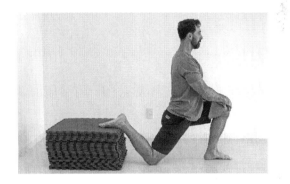

*Couch/Wall Hip Flexor Stretch – One Set of Thirty Seconds*

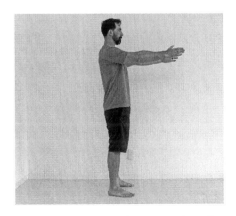 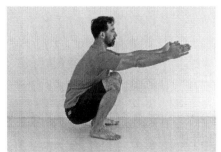

*Squats – One Set of Fifteen Repetitions*

Unfortunately, many of us find ourselves in prolonged sitting and standing postures due to our work activities. Even if you have a standing or adjustable desk, it is important to incorporate regular movement breaks to keep your body (and mind) healthy.

The exercises listed above can be performed in tight spaces, with the exception of the couch/wall hip flexor stretch. All of these exercises can be performed standing *or* sitting, so you can perform them in most work environments.

In an ideal situation, you should perform all of them every hour during your work day. However, we understand that this may not be possible for everyone. Most people who work eight-hour days only have one or two short breaks throughout the day. Fortunately, it only takes a few minutes to perform all of the exercises, thus allowing some people to briefly exercise at their desk or in their office without taking a formal "break" from their work. For those who are unable to perform all of these exercises several times throughout the day, know that even choosing one or two exercises to perform throughout the day will be very helpful and benefit not only your posture, but your state of mind and mental capacity.

Standing chin tucks and chair neck tilts will help relieve the built-up tension in your neck that is caused by prolonged static head positioning (which is very common among those who work in an office environment).

Thoracic extensions (with your elbows on the wall) will counteract your rounded-shoulder and head-forward (hunched) postures.

Finally, the squat exercise will get your blood moving and give your hips, knees, and ankles some needed motion after they have been still for a prolonged period of time.

# NECK/BACK EMPHASIS

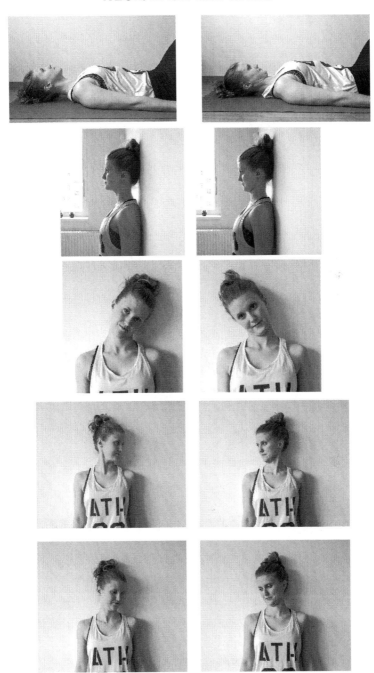

*Chin Tucks (Two Variations; Choose Two that are Appropriate for Your Level) – Two Sets of Ten Repetitions*

**Neck Strength (a neck extension and a neck flexion exercise variation that is appropriate for you) - 2 sets of 12 repetitions**

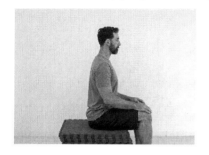 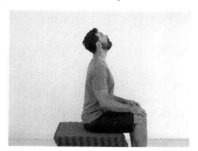

*Chair Neck Tilts*

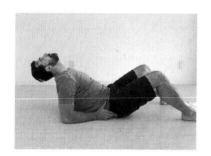 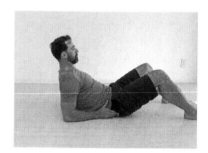

*Supine on Elbows Neck Flexion*

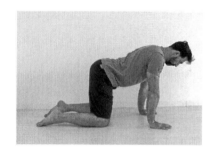 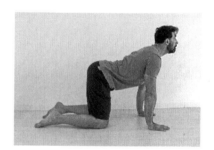

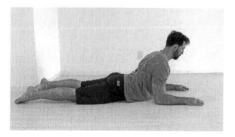 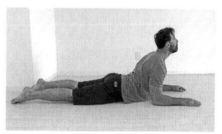

*Quadruped Neck Extension / Elbows Prone Neck Extension*

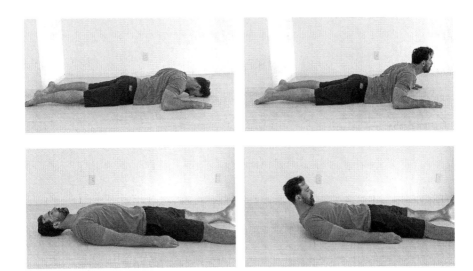

*Prone and Supine Bed or Table Neck Flexion and Extension*

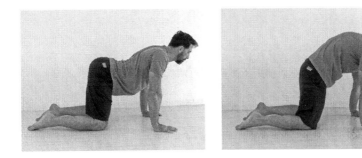

*Quadruped Cat/Camel –*
*Two Sets of Ten Repetitions*

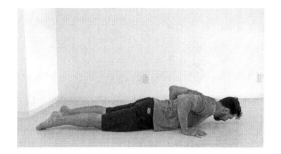 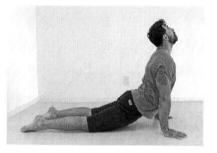

*Prone Extension Press –*
*Three Sets of Ten Repetitions*

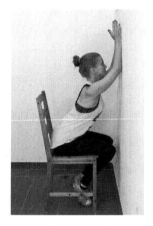 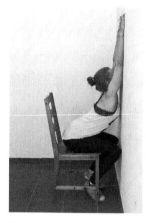

*Thoracic Extension (Elbows on Wall) –*
*Three Sets of Thirty Seconds*

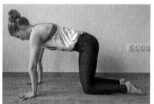 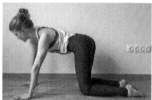 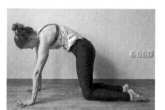

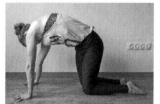 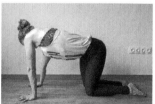 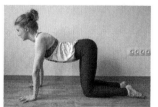

*Quadruped Spinal Circles – Two Sets of Ten Repetitions*

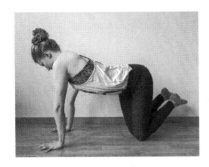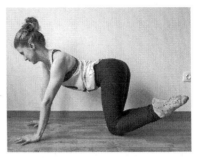

*Quadruped Spinal Sidebending –*
*Two Sets of Ten Repetitions*

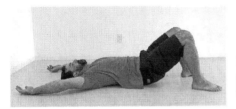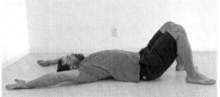

*Supine Hooklying Anterior and Posterior Pelvic Tilt –*
*Two Sets of Fifteen Repetitions*

This sequence emphasizes spinal exercises for mobility and strength/endurance. We tend to neglect our spines until we notice our neck and/or backs beginning to ache. Therefore, spending a training cycle devoted to this area is a great way to shore up our weaknesses and prevent future problems.

Choose two of the chin tuck exercise variations that work best for you. Begin with supine chin tucks and progress to the next variation if you feel they are too easy.

Choose one neck flexion and one neck extension exercise variation that is appropriate for your level of expertise.

Work on performing each exercise slowly and mindfully. This will give you room to notice any issues in your range of motion and anything else that needs improvement or refining. The end result is you will develop muscle control that leads to long-term retention of your mobility and flexibility gains.

## BACK/LOWER BODY EMPHASIS

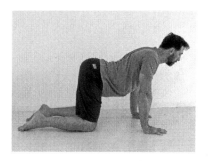 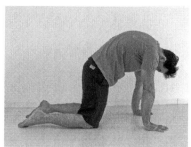

*Quadruped Cat/Camel –*
*Two Sets of Ten Repetitions*

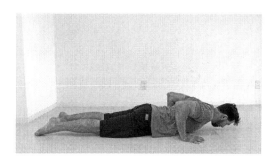 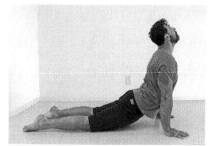

*Prone Extension Press –*
*Three Sets of Ten Repetitions*

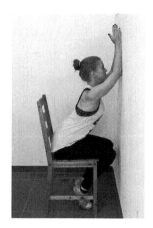 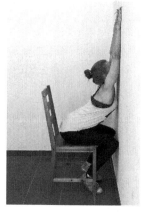

*Thoracic Extension (Elbows on Wall) –*
*Three Sets of Thirty Seconds*

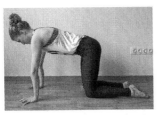 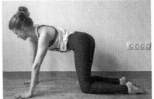 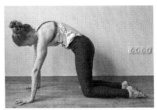

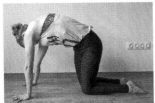 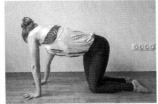 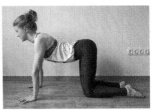

*Quadruped Spinal Circles —*
*Two Sets of Ten Repetitions*

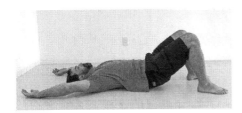 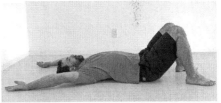

*Supine Hooklying Anterior and Posterior Pelvic Tilt —*
*Two Sets of Fifteen Repetitions*

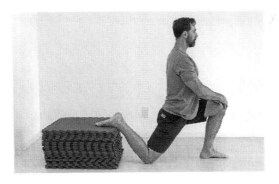

*Couch/Wall Hip Flexor Stretch — Three Sets of Thirty Seconds*

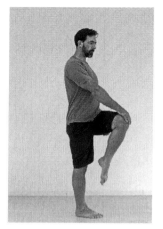 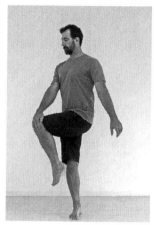

*Standing Hand-Resisted Hip Flexion (Appropriate Variation) –*
*Two Sets of Ten Repetitions*

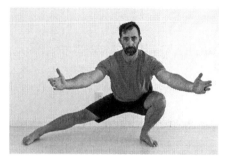 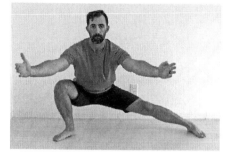

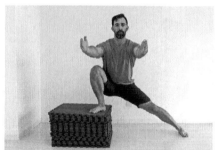 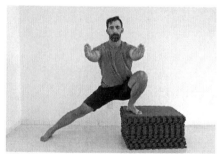

*Side-to-Side Squats – Two Sets of Twelve Repetitions*

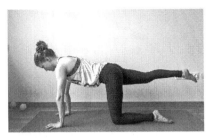
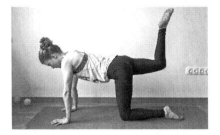
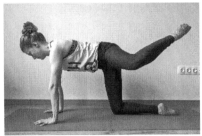
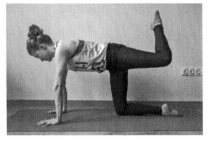

*Quadruped Kicks or Fire Hydrant – Three Sets of Ten Repetitions*

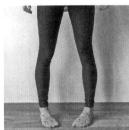
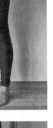
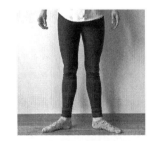

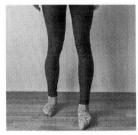
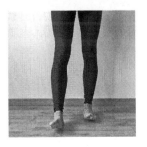
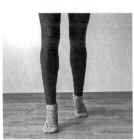

*Walking Foot Drills – One Set of Each Walk*

In this series of exercises, the emphasis on your back and lower body will tackle prevalent mobility restrictions in the back and lower limbs.

This routine begins with spinal mobility work in order to loosen up and bring awareness to this area. It then moves into the couch/wall hip flexor stretch and standing hand-resisted hip flexion (choose either the regular or rotating variation based on your ability level) exercises in order to prep for hip strength and endurance exercises.

Finally, the routine concludes with walking foot drills for your ankles and feet.

## MOVEMENT/RESET

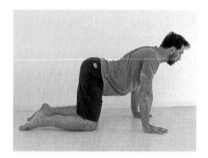 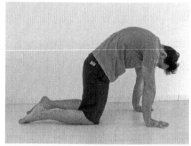

*Quadruped Cat/Camel – Two Sets of Ten Repetitions*

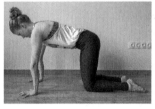 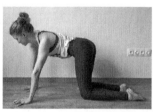 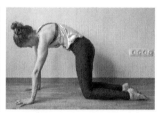

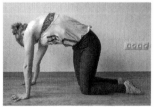 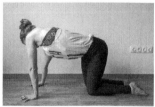 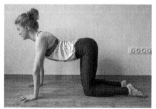

*Quadruped Spinal Circles – Two Sets of Ten Repetitions*

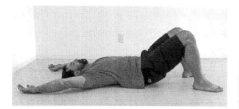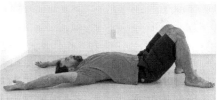

*Supine Hooklying Anterior and Posterior Pelvic Tilt –*
*Two sets of Fifteen Repetitions*

## Segmental Rolling – Three Repetitions of Each Roll

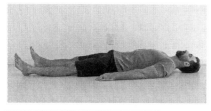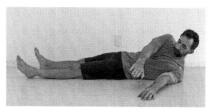
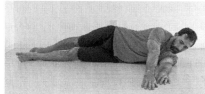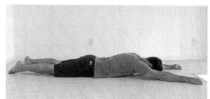

*Facing Up, Right Arm Roll*

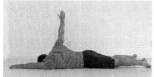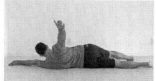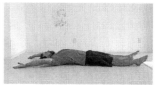

*Facing Down, Right Arm Roll*

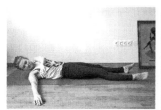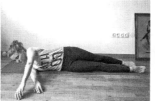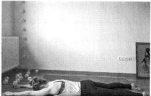

*Facing Up, Left Arm Roll*

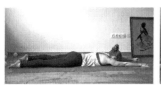 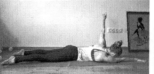 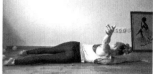

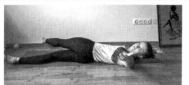 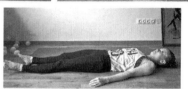

*Facing Down, Left Arm Roll*

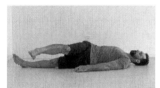 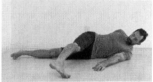 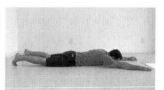

*Facing Up, Right Leg Roll*

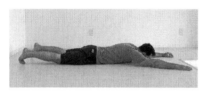 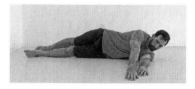

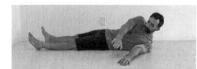 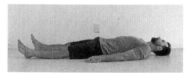

*Facing Down, Right Leg Roll*

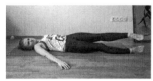 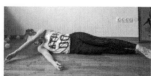 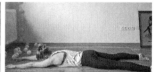

*Facing Up, Left Leg Roll*

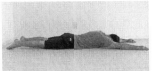 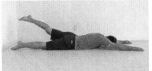 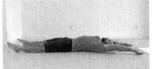

*Facing Down, Left Leg Roll*

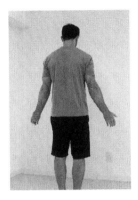 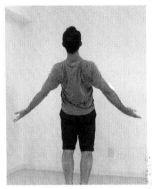

*Hyperextension Pose – Two Sets of Ten Repetitions*

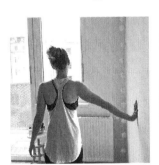 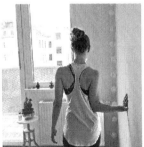 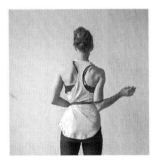

*Wall/Band Fix – Two Sets of Thirty Seconds*

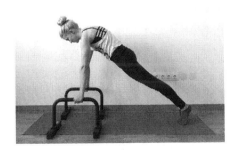 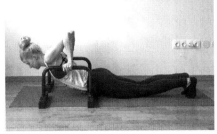

*Chair/Parallettes/Box Fix – Two Sets of Thirty Seconds*

This routine prioritizes mobility and the resets presented in this book. It works great as a comprehensive approach for reducing spinal tension and improving body awareness. The quadruped cat/camel, spinal circles, and pelvic tilts are good for complete spinal mobility, while segmental rolling integrates said mobility into full-body movements.

The resets, hyperextension pose, wall/band fix, and chair/parallettes/box fix are a good way to end your exercise session, as you have prepped your body with the previous movements and will be able to move into the exaggerated postures much more easily.

# ADD-ON PLANS FOR EXISTING ROUTINES

These two plans can be tacked on to your current training, either as separate sessions or as part of your training day. The first plan will focus on strength work, while the second plan will focus on mobility.

## STRENGTH

### Neck Strength (a neck extension and a neck flexion exercise variation that is appropriate for you) – Two Sets of Twelve Repetitions

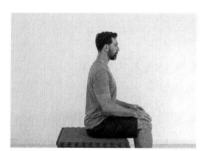 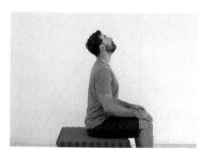

*Chair Neck Tilts*

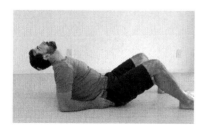 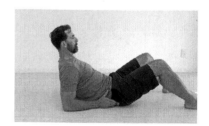

*Supine on Elbows Neck Flexion*

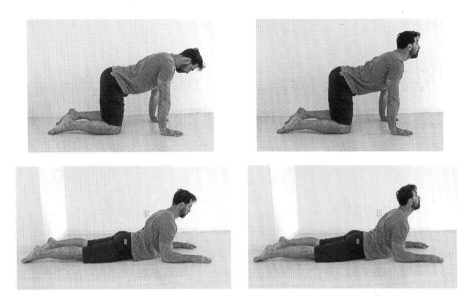

*Quadruped Neck Extension / Elbows Prone Neck Extension*

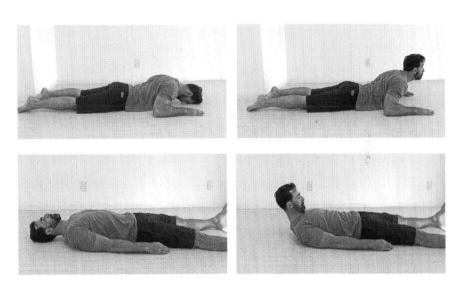

*Prone and Supine Bed or Table Neck Flexion and Extension*

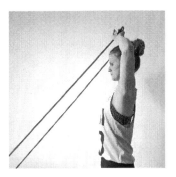

*Face Pulls – Three Sets of Twelve Repetitions*

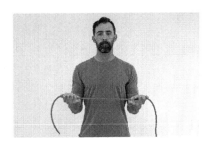 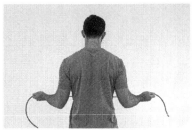

*Band External Rotation with Retraction – Three Sets of Twelve Repetitions*

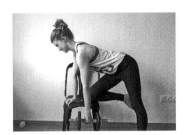 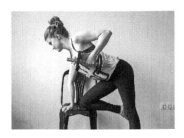

*Inverted Rows or One-Arm Dumbbell Rows –*
*Three Sets of Ten Repetitions*

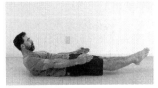 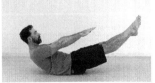 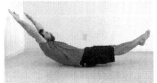

*Hollow Body Hold (the variation that is best for you) –*
*Three Sets of One Minute Holds*

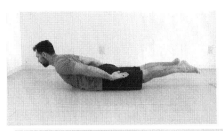
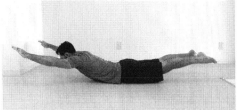
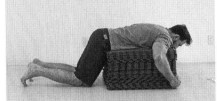
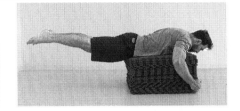

*Superman Hold or Reverse Hyperextension (the variation that is best for you) – Three Sets of One Minute Holds (or Twelve Repetitions)*

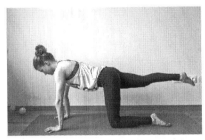
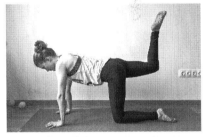
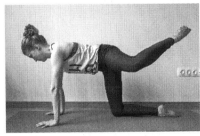
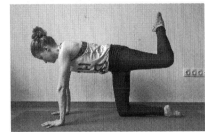

*Quadruped Kicks or Fire Hydrants – Three Sets of Twelve Repetitions*

This strengthening plan targets the primary areas that play a role in maintaining good postural alignment: your neck, upper back, abdominals, and glutes.

Choose one neck flexion and one neck extension exercise variation that is appropriate for your skill level.

# MOBILITY

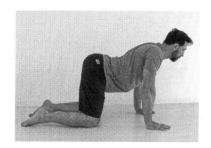 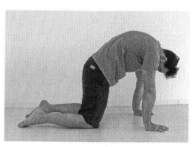

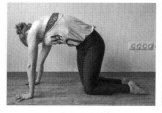 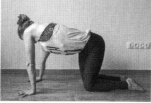 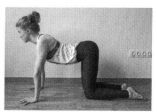

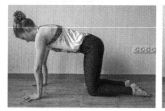 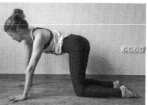 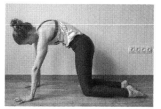

*Quadruped Cat/Camel or Quadruped Spinal Circles –
Three Sets of Ten Repetitions*

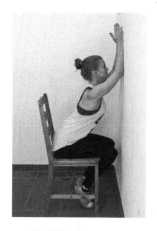 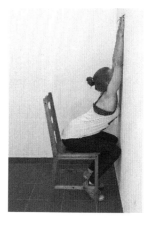

*Elbows on Wall Thoracic Extension – Three Sets of Thirty Seconds*

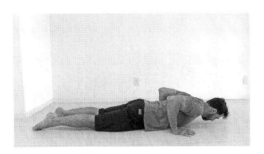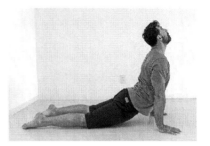

*Prone Extension Press – Three Sets of Ten Repetitions*

## Segmental Rolling – Three Repetitions of Each Roll

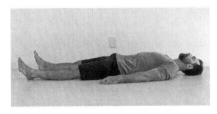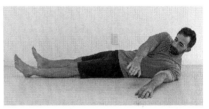
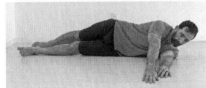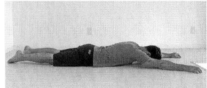

*Facing Up, Right Arm Roll*

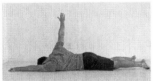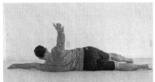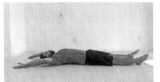

*Facing Down, Right Arm Roll*

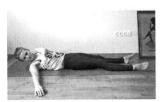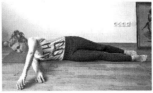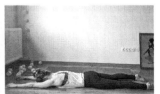

*Facing Up, Left Arm Roll*

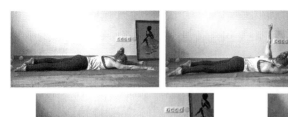
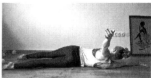
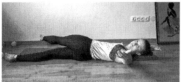
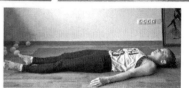

*Facing Down, Left Arm Roll*

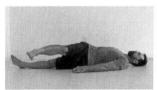
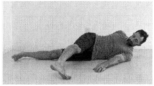
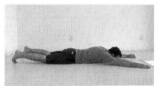

*Facing Up, Right Leg Roll*

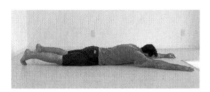
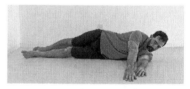
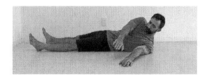
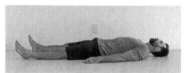

*Facing Down, Right Leg Roll*

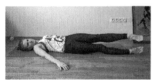
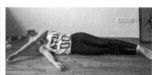
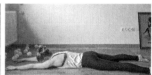

*Facing Up, Left Leg Roll*

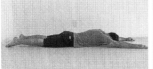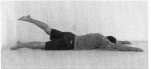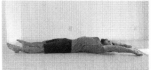

*Facing Down, Left Leg Roll*

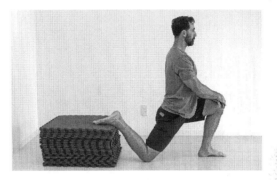

*Couch/Wall Hip Flexor Stretch – Three Sets of Thirty Seconds*

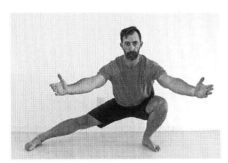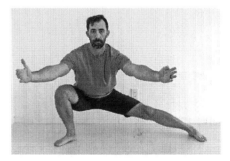

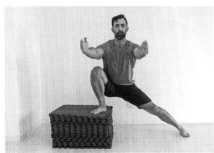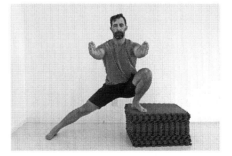

*Side-to-Side Squat – Three Sets of Twelve Repetitions*

The first three exercises of this mobility plan emphasize spinal mobility in areas that are commonly tight. You then integrate range-of-motion work with full-body segmental rolling movements before finishing with the couch/wall hip flexor stretch and side-to-side squat, which will increase mobility in your hips.

## CONNECT WITH US

systematicposture.com

stevenlow.org

gmb.io

# ABOUT THE AUTHORS

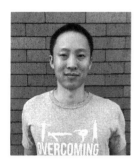 **Steven Low** is a former gymnast, coach, and the author of *Overcoming Gravity*. He has spent thousands of hours independently researching the scientific foundations of health, fitness and nutrition. His unique knowledge base enables him to offer numerous insights into practical care for injuries. Steven holds a Bachelor of Science in Biochemistry from the University of Maryland, College Park, as well as a Doctorate of Physical Therapy from the University of Maryland, Baltimore.

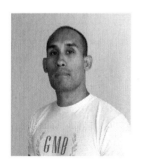 **Jarlo Ilano** has been a physical therapist (MPT) since 1998 and is a board certified orthopedic clinical specialist (OCS) with the American Board of Physical Therapy Specialties. He has had extensive postgraduate training in neck and back rehabilitation with an emphasis in manual therapy. He's been teaching martial arts for over 20 years and cofounded GMB Fitness to make strength and skill accessible so anyone can learn to move better and enjoy their lives.

# NOTES

1 Paul Ingraham, "Does Posture Correction Matter?," *PainScience.com*, 2004, www.painscience.com/articles/posture.php

2 Adam D. Galinsky; Li Huang, "How You Can Become More Powerful by Literally Standing Tall," *Scientific American*, January 4, 2011, www.scientificamerican.com/article/how-you-can-become-more-p/

3 Ohio State University, "Body Posture Affects Confidence in Your Own Thoughts," *Science Daily*, October 5, 2009, www.sciencedaily.com/releases/2009/10/091005111627.htm

4 Ibid.

5 Adam D. Galinsky; Li Huang, "How You Can Become More Powerful by Literally Standing Tall" and Vanessa Bohns; Scott S. Wiltermuth, "It hurts when I do this (or you do that): Posture and pain tolerance," *Journal of Experimental Social Psychology*, DOI: 10.1016/j.jesp.2011.05.022.

6 Adam D. Galinsky; Li Huang, "How You Can Become More Powerful by Literally Standing Tall."

7 Paul Ingraham, "Does Posture Correction Matter?"

8 RG Cohen; AN Vasavada; MM Wiest; M Schmitter-Edgecombe, "Mobility and Upright Posture Are Associated with Different Aspects of Cognition in Older Adults," *Frontiers in Aging Neuroscience*, DOI: 10.3389/fnagi.2016.00257.

9 V.L. Murrie; A.K. Dixon; W. Hollingworth; H. Wilson; T.A.C. Doyle, "Lumbar Lordosis: Study of Patients with and without Lower Back Pain," *Clinical Anatomy*, February 14, 2003, DOI: doi.org/10.1002/ca.10114 | G.F. Nakipoğlu; A. Karagöz; N. Ozgirgin, "The Biomechanics of the Lumbosacral Region in Acute and Chronic Lower Back Pain Patients," *Pain Physician*, July-August 2008 | Mohammad Reza Nourbakhsh; Amir Massoud Arab, "Relationship Between Mechanical Factors and Incidence of Low Back Pain," *Journal of Orthopaedic & Sports Physical Therapy*, 2002, DOI: 10.2519/jospt.2002.32.9.447

10  Mohammad Reza Nourbakhsh; Amir Massoud Arab, "Relationship Between Mechanical Factors and Incidence of Low Back Pain."

11  Paul Ingraham, "Does Posture Correction Matter?"

12  Ronald Melzack, "Pain and the Neuromatrix in the Brain," *Journal of Dental Education*, December 1, 2001, www.ncbi.nlm.nih.gov/pubmed/11780656

13  Robert J. Gatchel; Yuan Bo Peng; Madelon L. Peters; Perry N. Fuchs; Dennis C. Turk, "The Biopsychosocial Approach to Chronic Pain: Scientific Advances and Future Directions," *Psychological Bulletin*, July 2007, DOI: 10.1037/0033-2909.133.4.581

14  Adriaan Louw; Ina Diener; David S. Butler; Emilio J. Puentedura, "The Effect of Neuroscience Education on Pain, Disability, Anxiety, and Stress in Chronic Musculoskeletal Pain," *Archives of Physical Medicine and Rehabilitation*, 2011, DOI: 10.1016/j.apmr.2011.07.198 | Cormac G. Ryan; Heather G. Gray; Mary Newton; Malcolm H. Granat, "Pain Biology Education and Exercise Classes compared to Pain Biology Education Alone for Individuals with Chronic Lower Back Pain: A Pilot Randomised Controlled Trial," *Manual Therapy*, 2010, DOI: 10.1016/j.math.2010.03.003 | Lorimer Moseley; Michael K. Nicholas; Paul W. Hodges, "A Randomized Controlled Trial of Intensive Neurophysiology Education in Chronic Lower Back Pain," *The Clinical Journal of Pain*, 2004, DOI: 10.1097/00002508-200409000-00007

15  Bart W. Koes; Maurits van Tulder; Chung-Wei Christine Lin; Luciana G. Macedo; James McAuley; Chris Maher, "An Updated Overview of Clinical Guidelines for the Management of Non-Specific Lower Back Pain in Primary Care," *European Spine Journal*, December 2010, DOI: 10.1007/s00586-010-1502-y

16  Ibid.

17  Adrian C. Traeger; G. Lorimer Moseley; Markus Hübscher; other contributors, "Pain Education to Prevent Chronic Lower Back Pain: A Study Protocol for a Randomised Controlled Trial," *The BMJ*, June 2014, DOI: 10.1136/bmjopen-2014-005505

18  G. Lorimer Moseley; Alberto Gallace; Charles Spence, "Bodily Illusions in Health and Disease: Physiological and Clinical Perspectives and the Concept of a Cortical 'Body Matrix,'" *Neuroscience & Biobehavioral Reviews*, January 2012, DOI: 10.1016/j.neubiorev.2011.03.013

19  Erik Witvrouw; Nele Mahieu; Lieven Danneels; Peter McNair, "Stretching and Injury Prevention: An Obscure Relationship," *Sports Medicine*, 2004, www.ncbi.nlm.nih.gov/pubmed/15233597 | Lawrence Hart, "Effect of Stretching on Sport Injury Risk: A Review," *Clinical Journal of Sport Medicine*, 2005, www.ncbi.nlm.nih.gov/pubmed/15782063 | Christoffer Brushøj; Klaus Larsen; Elisabeth Albrecht-Beste;

Michael Bachmann Nielsen; Finn Løye; Per Hölmich, "Prevention of Overuse Injuries by a Concurrent Exercise Program in Subjects Exposed to an Increase in Training Load," *The American Journal of Sports Medicine*, 2008, DOI: 10.1177/0363546508315469 | Daniel Pereles; Alan Roth; Darby Thompson, "A Large, Randomized, Prospective Study of the Impact of a Pre-Run Stretch on the Risk of Injury in Teenage and Older Runners," *USA Track & Field*, www.usatf.org/stretchStudy/StretchStudyReport.pdf | Aviroop Biswas; Paul I. Oh; Guy E. Faulkner; and others, "Sedentary Time and its Association with Risk for Disease Incidence, Mortality, and Hospitalization in Adults," *Annals of Internal Medicine*, 2015, DOI: 10.7326/M14-1651

20 D. Czaprowski; P. Pawłowska; L. Stoliński; T. Kotwicki, "Active Self-correction of Back Posture in Children Instructed with 'Straighten your Back' Command," *Manual Therapy*, October 2014; DOI: 10.1016/j.math.2013.10.005

21 D. Czaprowski; P. Pawłowska; A. Kolwicz-Gańko; D. Sitarski; A. Kedra, "The Influence of the 'Straighten your Back' Command on the Sagittal Spinal Curvatures in Children with Generalized Joint Hypermobility," *BioMed Research International*, January 2017, DOI: 10.1155/2017/9724021

22 Dr. Vladimir Janda, "Janda's Crossed Syndromes," *JandaApproach.com*, accessed January 27, 2017, www.jandaapproach.com/the-janda-approach/jandas-syndromes

23 Eun-Kyung Kim; Jin Seop Kim, "Correlation between Rounded Shoulder Posture, Neck Disability Indices, and Degree of Head-forward Posture," *Journal of Physical Therapy Science*, October 2016, DOI: 10.1589/jpts.28.2929 | John Manor; Elizabeth Hibberd; Meredith Petschauer; Joseph Myers, "Acute Effects of Posture Shirts on Rounded-shoulder and Forward-head Posture in College Students," *Journal of Sport Rehabilitation*, December 2016, DOI: 10.1123/jsr.2014-0304

24 Mark Lepper; D. Greene; R. Nisbett, "Undermining Children's Intrinsic Interest with Extrinsic Reward: A Test of the 'Overjustification' Hypothesis," October 1973.

25 E. McAuley; K.S. Courneya, D.L. Rudolph; C.L. Lox, "Enhancing Exercise Adherence in Middle-Aged Males and Females," *Preventive Medicine*, 1994, DOI: 10.1006/pmed.1994.1068 | C.E. Matthews; S.M. George; S.C. Moore; and others, "Amount of Time Spent in Sedentary Behaviors and Cause-specific Mortality in US Adults," *The American Journal of Clinical Nutrition*, 2012, DOI: 10.3945/ajcn.111.019620 | Earl S. Ford; Carl J. Caspersen, "Sedentary Behaviour and Cardiovascular Disease: A Review of Prospective Studies," *International Journal of Epidemiology*, 2012, DOI: 10.1093/ije/dys078

*Additional references are listed at the end of each chapter.*

Made in the USA
Middletown, DE
06 August 2018